Textbook of Sport for the Disabled

This book is dedicated to all those disabled men, women and youngsters whose courage, tenacity and skill have proved to society that disability is no barrier to achievement in high class sport.

"You are the living demonstration of the marvels of the virtue of energy. You have given a great example, which We would like to emphasize, because it can be a lead to all: you have shown what an energetic soul can achieve, in spite of apparently insurmountable obstacles imposed by the body."

Pope John XXIII, at the International Stoke Mandeville Games in Rome, 1960.

Textbook
of
Sport for the Disabled

Professor Sir Ludwig Guttmann CBE FRS

MD FRCP FRCS Hon FRCP(C) Hon DSc Hon DChir Hon LLD

Founder and former Director, National Spinal Injuries Centre, Stoke Mandeville Hospital, Aylesbury, Bucks; Director, Stoke Mandeville Sports Stadium for the Paralysed and other Disabled; Founder-President, International Stoke Mandeville Games Federation; Founder-President, British Sports Association for the Multi-Disabled; President, International Sports Organisation of the Disabled.

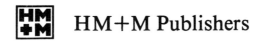 HM+M Publishers

GLG DE

First English Edition
Published by HM+M Publishers Ltd.
Milton Road, Aylesbury, Bucks, England

0 85602 055 9

Printed in Great Britain at the Alden Press, Oxford

Contents

Preface

There has been a dynamic approach in recent years in this country to the long-term development of sport in all its forms for both able-bodied and physically handicapped athletes. The moving forces, so far as the disabled are concerned, have been the Chronically Sick and Disabled Persons Act 1971, introduced by Alfred Morris MP, and the active support given to the development of sport amongst the disabled by the Sports Council and the Central Council of Physical Recreation.

It is an unfortunate fact that the sporting activities of the disabled have been largely ignored, or at best mentioned only briefly, in the many books available on sport and recreation for the able-bodied; there is, therefore, a great demand for a comprehensive textbook on sport for the disabled in the English Language. I have been urged and encouraged by many friends—teachers, physiotherapists, physical instructors, coaches, referees, administrators, members of the medical profession, and disabled sportsmen alike—to write such a book, in view of my experience gained during the last 30 years.

The types of disability discussed in this book are amputation, blindness, cerebral palsy, deafness and spinal paralysis, as these are the conditions which are already covered by special sports organisations. It is logical and natural that the underlying principles, techniques and rules relating to the sporting activities suited to those who suffer from such physical handicaps should be applied in future to other forms of disablement.

Emphasis has been given to a detailed survey of sport for spinal paraplegics and tetraplegics, in view of the fact that sport for this category was an entirely new development. Started during the last World War, this sports movement has made outstanding progress and has developed into a world-wide organisation.

Research over many years into the various aspects of sport for disabled persons has resulted in many discoveries which have been applied to the practical management of their sporting activities, and standards of performance have been statistically evaluated to prepare the ground for the further development of skill in individual sports.

Sports for the disabled, as with the able-bodied, must have agreed rules, enforced by those responsible for the management and organisation of sports events. Moreover, such rules must necessarily be combined with correct classification according to the extent of physical deficit to ensure fair play, and such classifications have been compiled over the years in co-operation with panels of medical and technical experts of ISMGF and ISOD in the various fields of disablement. Therefore, it seemed to be essential to include in this book at least the main internationally-accepted rules, which largely follow the rules of sport for the able-bodied but are, naturally, adjusted to suit the disabled.

Special attention has also been paid to giving details of the physical, psychological and social effects which sport exerts on the disabled sportsmen, women and children.

I have been greatly assisted in the establishment of this book by Miss Joan Scruton MBE and Mr. Charlie Atkinson, who from the beginning have been my closest co-workers in the development of sport for the paralysed and other disabled. I have also been most fortunate in having with me through the years a team of enthusiastic coaches, officials and many volunteers.

I have been very fortunate in receiving a grant for secretarial help from the National Fund for Research into Crippling Diseases which I have very much appreciated.

Mrs. Kate Lambrechts has been of invaluable help in typing and preparing the manuscript, and I also appreciate the excellent work of Mr. Derek Stanton, the photographer at Stoke Mandeville Hospital.

Finally, my warmest thanks are due to my publishers, Mr. Peter Medcalf, Mr. John Medcalf and the editor, Mr. Patrick West, for their understanding of and compliance with my wishes.

I hope this book will be of service and guidance to all concerned with sport for our disabled fellow-men, and especially for the sportsmen and sportswomen themselves, and that it will prove a useful contribution to the history of sport in general.

Stoke Mandeville
January 1976   LUDWIG GUTTMANN

1

Reflections on Sport in General

Terminology and Definition of Sport

The basic ideas of sport and its interpretation (the word originates from the Latin word *disportare*) have been expressed in the world literature by a number of definitions, varying from concise, dictionary descriptions to detailed, complex and sometimes verbose technical, sociological and philosophical interpretations. It is beyond the scope of this book to go into a detailed analysis of the phenomenon of sport as discussed by contemporary writers, such as Coubertin (1949), Bouet (1968, 1969), Diem (1942, 1950, 1957, 1960), Dufrenne (1950), Huizinga (1949), Jokl (1965), Kaplan (1968), Loy (1969), Lüschen (1960, 1970), McIntosh (1963), Slusher (1973), Wenkart (1963), Weiss (1969) and others, but a few examples may be given which reveal the different interpretations. In 1962 K. Widener in *Erziehung heute—Erziehung für morgen* (Education today—Education for tomorrow) gave the following definition: "We understand by sport that part of the body culture by which, through rhythmic and forceful activities, physical and mental functions such as intelligence, reactions, body awareness, kinesthetics, etc., are required. These activities are expressed in *Strahlbedeutung* and *Diensibedeutung*, whereby differentiated changes in process are possible. In all sports events, action is more important than result". The two specially devised new terms in the German language—*Strahlbedeutung* and *Dienstbedeutung*—are rather ambiguous and difficult to understand, and one may ask whether such definitions really help the proper understanding of the phenomenon of sport. A different though somewhat circumstantial interpretation has recently been given by Lüschen (1970): "Sport is non-representative, competitive activity in interaction with other persons. It is primarily based on physical skill. It carries with it intrinsic and extrinsic rewards. The amount of extrinsic rewards (material and/or social) determines where, on a continuum between play and work, a specific sport activity is located."

Sport has also been defined by UNESCO as "Any physical activity which has the character of play and which involves a struggle with oneself or with others, or a confrontation with natural elements is sport. If this activity involves competition it must be performed with a spirit of sportsmanship. There can be no true sport without fair play. All rules must be observed with this in mind."

In contrast, the German dictionary (Duden) defines sport briefly as "Spiel und Leibesübungen (play and physical exercise)", while the Oxford dictionary defines sport as "fun" and "diversion". Whether one accepts or not the views of philologists that the English word 'sport' is derived from the old French word 'esporter', this is of lesser importance than its definition, which means "to amuse oneself by physical exercise". This definition of sport, which incorporates recreation as a basic principle, has a special meaning in our modern society of technology, with it, continuing progress of mechanisation on the one hand and steady increase in leisure hours on the other. Leisure can be used for cultural activities such as art, crafts etc., but we are here concerned with physical exercise as one of the pursuits of leisure.

Sport and Recreation in Modern Society

Sport has many functions and can be enjoyed in various ways; it can be classified as follows:

Passive Spectator Sport

Throughout the centuries millions of people in every country have taken a passive attitude towards sport and this still prevails on an even larger scale in our modern technological society. It applies to both the able-bodied and the physically handicapped sections of the community, who enjoy the sport of others by attending their spectacular sporting events, in particular soccer, rugby, professional wrestling, athletics, baseball or ice-hockey matches, or by following them in front of their television sets. This passive approach to sport serves both as pastime and leisure, as well as a means of social contact, and not only as an enjoyable entertainment to get away from the stresses of daily life, to relieve boredom and frustration and to escape from the monotony of repetitive work; but for many it is also an emotional outlet. In this connection circus-sport shows are another form of spectator sport. For young people spectator sport is often an outlet for their restlessness and aggressiveness which, alas, all too often results in loss of self-control and degenerates into the rowdyism which in recent years has taken such ugly forms, particularly at soccer matches and has forced the authorities concerned to take stern preventive measures. Moreover, an important sideline of spectator sport for many people is the opportunity it provides for gambling, which, particularly in horse or dog racing (in eastern countries, cock-fighting) has become enormously popular and has been exploited commercially on a vast scale.

Active Sport

This form of sport, with which we are concerned in this book, can conveniently be divided into:

(a) *Performance (Leistungs) Sport.* This is competitive sport, aimed at increasing the standard of performance, if possible to the highest level. (High Performance, (Höchstleistung) Sport. Although top-standard performance will always be confied to a select group of specially-gifted people there is no doubt that the average standard of performance has increased steadily commensurate with improved sports facilities and improved techniques of training and coaching, and this applies today as much to the disabled as it does to the able-bodied. For instance, the introduction of the fibreglass pole and the foam rubber landing cushion has greatly improved the standard of performance of pole-vaulting by the able-bodied just as the introduction of the modern fibreglass bow with its stabilising antennae and adjustable sights has improved the technique and performance of archery by both able-bodied and wheelchair archers. Not only is competitive sport possible between individuals or teams, but it can also be carried out in isolation in combat with oneself in certain sports such as archery, pistol shooting, skating, running and others. In competitive sport agreed rules are indispensable to ensure fair play, and it will be shown later how important rules also are in sport for the disabled, especially in wheelchair basketball. Moreover, unlike their able-bodied colleagues, there is need for the proper classification of disabled sportsmen and women according to their physical, and in cerebral palsy also mental, deficit.

(b) *Recreational-Leisure Sport.* Although it would be quite wrong to deny the great recreational value of competitive sport, it is the non-competitive leisure sport which provides health-giving exercise and has recreation as its primary aim. There is a wealth of non-competitive sports ranging from tranquil angling or hiking to tough and strenuous activities such as rock climbing, squash and surf-riding. It may be stressed, however, that the usual distinction between non-competitive leisure sport and competitive performance sport is only of relative significance, for many competitive sports, such as swimming, riding, squash, and running are used as leisure activities, and vice versa, most leisure sports such as snooker, bowling, riding, angling, swimming, croquet, sailing, and others are included in competitive sport. Although dancing is certainly a very popular pastime and leisure activity, whether it can be considered as a sport is still a matter of conjecture. It is true that dancing is undertaken competitively by dancing clubs in national and international contests, but this also applies to other pastime and leisure activities such as chess, dominoes, etc. without their being considered as sport in the true sense of the word.

(c) *Adventure Sport*. Although many sports contain an element of risk, there are some in which the degree of risk is high and these often appeal to people who find less dangerous individual or team sports unattractive. Adventure sports include rock-climbing and Alpine mountaineering, parachuting, flying, gliding (hang-gliding), certain athletics, motor racing both in cars and motor cycles, surf-riding and Alpine skiing (this especially for disabled persons such as amputees and the blind), diving into rivers, lakes and the sea without first ascertaining the depth of the water, and also sub-aqua diving. Although these sports provide profound satisfaction in mastering difficult techniques and dangerous situations and environments, without doubt they cause very severe injuries and many deaths every year. It may be noted that diving into shallow water ranks high amongst the causes of injuries of the cervical spinal cord, as a result of fractures of the cervical spine. It is a tragedy that these accidents mainly affect young people, especially those aged between 17 and 25 years, who are transformed by such an injury in a nick of a second from a healthy individual into a helpless physical wreck of a tetraplegic for life. The warnings I have given for many years in my lectures and writings to the able-bodied not to dive into rivers and lakes of unknown depth or into rough seas with high waves are still valid. Education can help to diminish these tragedies, and it should be undertaken in school, as well as by instructors at swimming pools, just as systematically as is the education of youngsters in road safety and in the prevention of accidents.

There are some individuals who in spite of a severe disability sustained during their adventure sport, are nevertheless so irresistibly attracted to this type of sport that they resume their particular sport or take up a similar one. For example, an Australian sportsman from Adelaide became a spinal paraplegic in a kite crash. After discharge from hospital he became interested in hang-gliding and built his own hang-glider, adjusted to his paraplegia. At the time of writing he had made 25 flights, reaching heights of 150 metres, and is now president of the South Australian Hang-Glider Association. "The sound of sail flapping and the wind in the rigging," he says, "is music to me".

(d) *Clinical-Remedial Sport*. Sport as remedial exercise has a long history (see Chapter 3 on historical background). During and after the first World War sporting activities were used in the treatment of amputees and the blind. However, it was not until the second World War that sporting activities as part of clinical management were introduced into the rehabilitation of patients who were paraplegic and tetraplegic as a result of spinal cord injuries.

The immense value of sport in the physical, psychological and social rehabilitation of these most severely physically handicapped patients was recognised and became the incentive to many of them to carry on with their sporting activities after discharge from hospital and to become true sportsmen and sportswomen in their own right. Clinical sport is now widely used and has gained its secure place in the field of sport. Details will be discussed in the appropriate parts of this book.

Sociological Aspects of Sport and Recreation

Recreational activities in one way or another are playing an ever-increasing part in the life of the individual, as well as of society as a whole, in this and many other countries. Consequently, the demand for greater variety in recreation and more adequate facilities for sport has dramatically increased in recent years, and this applies today as much to the disabled as it does to the able-bodied in the community, including school-leavers and the elderly. Both the Sports Council and the Central Council for Physical Recreation have done much in Great Britain in recent years to meet these demands.

In analysing the driving forces which have unleashed the pressure of demands on local, regional and governmental authorities to provide more and better recreational facilities, one has to consider a combination of medical, social and economic factors.

(a) Growth of Population

Statistics of the Registrar General for 1968 revealed an increase in the population of this country of about 3 million and a further increase of 3.5 million was forecast for the next decade. It is true that this increase affects mainly the South of England, but it applies not only to the larger cities but also to smaller towns. For instance, the population of Aylesbury almost doubled from 21,050 in 1951 to 40,569 in 1971, and that of High Wycombe (both are in Buckinghamshire) increased from 40,702 in 1951 to 59,340 in 1971. The population of the county of Buckinghamshire increased during that period from 386,291 to 578,559.

This population explosion has created a situation of more people living in a more constricted space in blocks of flats in high buildings with infinitely less garden space available. It applies to young and old people alike, thanks to greatly reduced infant mortality and the increased life expectancy of people over 60 years of age. Moreover, it also applies to the 3 million disabled people in this country. Because of the great advances made since the last World War in medical management and social, professional and industrial rehabilitation, the life span even of the most severely disabled people, such as spinal cord paraplegics and tetraplegics, has enormously increased and in many cases may not be materially different from that of the able-bodied. Continuous immigration also contri-

butes to the over-all increase of the population.

(b) The Effects of Automation on Working life

The rapid progress of technology and industry in our technocratic society in the last 20 years or so has created more automation of production. Work, which only a few years ago had to be carried out by sometimes hundreds of workers, can now be done by machines with only a few workers in attendance. However, one has to remember that industrial work has become more and more repetitive, and in the long run the monotony of automation may have the adverse psychological effect on the worker of creating boredom, resulting in frustration. To counteract frustration, there is an increased desire, often unconscious, for recreative activity to preserve or promote interest and enjoyment in life.

(c) Increased Leisure Time

In step with the automation of production has come a reduction in basic working hours, which have decreased from 45 in 1961 to 40 hours or less and, since 1968, for industrial workers to 38 hours and even to three to four days' work per week. Overtime working has also considerably decreased. It must also be remembered that, according to statistics, the length of paid annual holidays has increased for both manual and office workers (Reports Nos. 110, 1963, and 134, 1966, of The Industrial Society), which also leaves more time for recreational activities. The holiday industry has taken great advantage of this, as evidenced by the enormous flood of advertisements which appear almost daily on television and in the press. Moreover, Great Britain and other countries are at present hit by increasing inflation, resulting in steadily rising unemployment and the consequent enforced inactivity of thousands of people. Here sporting activities can relieve frustration and apathy at least to some extent.

(d) Raised Standard of Living

There is no doubt that, with the increase of

wages and salaries to which overtime work makes an essential contribution, the living standards of the working population have gone up significantly, and an expression of this is undoubtedly the tremendous growth of car ownership during the last 10 years. It may be noted that, according to surveys by the Automobile Association, a greater percentage of car owners are using their cars for non-business purposes, which facilitates greatly their participation in recreative activities. It also means that people walk less and, therefore, there is all the more need for various forms of active exercise.

(e) Changes in Education

It is a far cry from the days of child labour—nearly a century ago—to the present attitude of society towards the education of children and youngsters. There was no time in those by-gone days for recreation by play and games, but only for rest to recover from fatigue, exhaustion and the frustration of work. Physical education and recreation have received considerable recognition in schools, and since World War II the Ministry of Education has provided large playing fields around schools, which have replaced the confined playgrounds between school buildings of the past. With the raising of the school leaving age and the development of higher education for a great number of youngsters on the one hand and the increasing difficulties of job-finding in a time of inflation on the other, the need for recreational facilities through sport is still rising for this section of the community. There is now an increasing number of swimming pools in schools; moreover, for schools which do not have their own pools, education departments of local authorities have arranged regular swimming sessions for their pupils in nearby public swimming pools. Thus, ever since the opening of the Stoke Mandeville Sports Stadium for the Paralysed and other Disabled in 1969, bus-loads of school children from neighbouring schools come every morning for swimming lessons, and on certain days the Sports Hall of the Stadium is used by school

children in the afternoon for badminton. There is now a wider range of physical activities available in schools and colleges for both able-bodied and disabled pupils. Even special schools for physically and mentally handicapped children have their own facilities for sporting activities.

The Rôle of Sport in Recreational Activities

Thus, sport in one form or another is today generally accepted by modern society as one of the most popular means of recreation. This is no doubt largely due to a better understanding of both the physical and psychological values of sport, but on the other hand, from all that has been said in the foregoing paragraphs, it is clear that sport has become a national need for sociological reasons. Sport, in particular competitive team sport, today plays an essential part in directing the increased leisure time of young and old into the proper channels. For the young, sport and play represent a natural outlet for abundant energy and their natural competitive and aggressive instincts. Moreover, at least for some individuals, it helps to build character by promoting certain moral qualities. The author agrees with the view held by those who contend that to some extent delinquency among young people is the result of boredom and lack of opportunity or desire for suitable physical activity. The misguided and misfired energy of some youngsters all too often deteriorates into hooliganism and criminal behaviour, and the destructive activities of 'mods and rockers', 'Hell's angels' and various types of 'angry brigades' have been a serious nuisance to society at large for some time. One can, therefore, wholeheartedly support the following recommendation, made some years ago in the report of the Wolfenden Committee on Sport and the Community (page 107): "More should be done to ensure that young people in their last months at school and their first months at work are well informed about the opportunities open to them in the field of sport." If the Wolfenden Committee had paid so much attention to the needs of the disabled (which were not mentioned in the report at all despite the Committee's attention being drawn to that ever-increasing section of the community), we would have been much more advanced in providing proper facilities for the disabled than we are today.

However, it must be noted that there is no statistical evidence as to whether or not engagement in sport constitutes a means of preventing delinquency. Since in recent years penal institutions and welfare organisations have used sport as a way of socially rehabilitating delinquents, this might give opportunities for the study of this interesting problem in more detail. It cannot be said either that engagement in sport represents, in principle, a barrier to violence. In fact, as mentioned before, there are certain sports, such as boxing, professional wrestling, soccer, baseball, and rugby football, which tend to promote violence amongst both players and spectators. However, these excesses, which by education and stricter control could be greatly diminished, cannot outweigh the overall benefits of sport.

Age and Sport

There is really no age-limit for active participation in sport, and its value is becoming increasingly recognised even amongst people of advancing years, judging from the greatly increased interest in various forms of sport, in particular indoor bowling by 'senior citizens'. Ageing, with its degenerative changes in the organism, is a natural developmental process in man as well as in animals, but there is some evidence that at least premature ageing of civilized man can be slowed down, if not prevented, by continuing mental and physical activity. There is abundant evidence of people in ancient and modern times who, in spite of old age, remained active in various sports such as running, mountaineering and skiing, even achieving high performance. Carl Diem (1957) wrote an interesting survey on this subject in a paper *Sport and Age*, delivered at the 18th Congress of German Sports Medicine. An unusually outstanding sportsman in this

respect in this century was the late King Gustav V of Sweden, who only a short time before his death at the age of 92 was still able to take part in tennis tournaments. In view of the modern trend to encourage people of advanced age to engage in sporting activities, it is perhaps timely to quote Cicero, the famous ancient Roman writer who in his paper, *Cato major de senectute*, gave a most appropriate summing-up of his views, which corresponds very well with the modern approach towards old age: "pugnandum tam quam contra morbem sic contra senectutem—one must fight old age like a disease!"

It is interesting to discover the percentage of both able-bodied and disabled athletes who still compete in international sports competitions beyond the age of 35. A recent statistic compiled in 1975 (*Lancet*, 1975) of competitors in the Olympic Games over the age of 35 revealed only 17 per cent. A survey of the 280 registered competitors in the 1974 National Stoke Mandeville Games for the Paralysed, shows that 28.5 per cent. were over the age of 35, ie. 35 to 50, and in the 1974 International Stoke Mandeville Games, out of 538 registered competitors 22.5 per cent. were over 35; of these, 11.3 per cent. were between the ages of 35 and 40 and 11.2 per cent. between 40 and 50. While Olympic athletes over the age of 35 took part almost entirely in competitions like sailing and other events which do not entail great muscular effort, in both the National and International Stoke Mandeville Games competitors of well over 35 still took part in field and track events, table tennis, swimming, weight-lifting and even basketball, and in the last event 9.7 per cent. were over 35. This clearly shows that disabled sportsmen and women are definitely anxious to continue their competitive sporting activities into middle and later age.

Sport and the Arts

Some years ago, the author had the opportunity to watch two outstanding representatives of the arts in the performance of their work. One was the late Sir James Gunn, R.A., while working on a portrait. It was fascinating to observe the delicate and economically graded movements of the fingers and hand muscles in relation to the posture of his arm, trunk and legs. These delicate gradations of localized muscular contractions were as intimately bound up with the sense of touch as those of a skilled neurosurgeon operating on the brain or spinal cord. The other artist was Dame Margot Fonteyn during her performance in *Romeo and Juliet*, exposing a different and infinitely more dynamic type of superb mastery of precision and co-ordination of rhythmic movements of all parts of the body. These movements were not merely mechanical in form, time and space, but were a self-expression of a means of transmitting an idea. Different as the pattern of movement of these two artists may have been, it was the complete understanding of the body—ie the creative awareness of neuromuscular co-ordination—which was the common feature of the beauty of their physical performance.

This experience, more than anything which the author had previously learned about the physiology of movement, convinced him of the close link which exists between the beauty of the arts and the beauty of sport. Sport, too, can combine perfection of physical performance with beauty. To give one example: anyone who watched the refinement and grace of the competitors—particularly the females—when performing difficult gymnastic feats on parallel bars or trapeze at the Olympic Games in Tokyo, Mexico or Munich will readily agree that such beautiful performances can only be accomplished by systematic training; training which results in complete understanding of both the muscular strength and the co-ordination of the locomotor system of the body as the determining factor in the formation of an artistic pattern of movement—whereby that pattern of movement becomes automatic in the achievement of perfect execution and top performance. The author experienced the same sensation during the Olympiades of the Paralysed in Israel and Heidelberg, when watching the underwater movements of paralysed swimmers through glass. The beauty of sport was well recognised in ancient times, and the preservation of its interpretation in sculpture is indeed an eternal documentation of the understanding of the beauty of pattern-formation in the human body by ancient masters.

Sport and Ethics

Today sport plays an ever-increasing integral part in the life of the individual, as it does in the life of nations, and represents as much a positive element in the culture of our modern life as it did in the culture of ancient nations. It must be remembered that physical education in ancient times was of a religious nature, and the sports festivals of ancient nations, whether in Asia or Greece, were based on ethical principles dedicated to the gods. There is still something of this left in the sports performances of Asiatic nations. If one watches both amateur and professional Japanese wrestling one cannot but be greatly impressed by the disciplined ceremonial rules accompanying this sport. Even professional wrestling tournaments were carried out with chivalry and respect for the judge and opponent and had nothing of that brutality combined with clownery which is sometimes demonstrated by our western style of professional wrestling, as can be seen on television, where that sport may deteriorate into farce. This may be quite amusing as entertainment but has little resemblance to the fine sport of amateur wrestling.

Sport and Politics

It was significant of the ethical attitude of the founders of the ancient Olympic Games that they placed these Games under the authority of Zeus Philios, the god of Friendship. Only when the concept of friendship, chivalry and respect for the competitor in sporting activities was replaced by violence, national chauvinism and commercialism were the Olympic Games doomed to failure, resulting in their inglorious conclusion. The decadent athleticism with its brutal form of sport found its expression in the gladiatorial competitions in ancient Rome. It is regrettable that sport in our society, and not only professional sport, is not free from commercialism, and the interference of money in sports performance must lead both to deterioration in the ideals of sport and to corruption.

The cultural values of sport were revived by Pierre de Coubertin (1894, 1922), the founder of the modern Olympic Games—but alas, there is still a long way to go before his philosophy of the ethics of sport becomes the dominating factor in our, at present, highly mechanized Olympic Games, fraught with political and racial biases, as demonstrated in the Olympic Games in Mexico and, in particular, in 1972 in Munich. These tragic events clearly dispel the myth that sport helps international understanding. So long as national or international sports organisations bow to political systems, whatever they may be, sport will still be exploited for political aims. In view of the continuing increase of international contests, the development of exaggerated nationalistic attitudes and chauvinism should be resisted as being most detrimental to the ideals of sport. Surely the outrageous chauvinistic behaviour of certain sportsmen during the Olympic Games in Mexico and Munich must bring home to the various nations how serious political involvement in sport has become! If any lessons were to be learned from the tragic events in Munich—starting with the expulsion of the Rhodesian Team as a result of the Olympic Committee's submission to political pressure and culminating in the massacre of the Israeli Team—they are that national, racial and religious prejudices and politics must be firmly and radically banned from sport. In this connection it was a fundamental step forward in restoring true sportsmanship, unity and friendship amongst nations when the South African Government just recently deviated from their racial segregative policies, at least for the international sports festival of the International Stoke Mandeville Games for the Paralysed, by allowing for the first time a multi-racial team of coloured and white sportsmen to participate in the 1975 Olympics for the Paralysed, the competitors being selected on merit only. This breakthrough in the apartheid problem, achieved in sport of the paralysed and other disabled, has recently been enlarged to sport in general.

Man can only hope that this decision of the South African Government to abandon apartheid in sport may produce the appropriate reactions in the Olympic Committee as well as in other international sports organisations to free sport from political pressure and prejudices of race, creed and colour, and to restore the Olympic Games to their original ideals.

Sport and Personality

Interest in personality problems in sport has been greatly intensified, commensurate with the development of psychology and psycho-analysis. A considerable number of experimental psychological techniques, including even hypnosis, has been employed for the assessment of personality features in athletes in various types of sport, in particular for the study of their motivations. However, it must be remembered that these studies were made under certain experimental conditions and circumstances, and therefore, although differences were found in certain mental attitudes, such as aggression, anxiety, neurasthenia or hypochondriacal behaviour, between athletes and non-athletes or between athletes in various types of sports, the results cannot be generalized. An excellent survey of these methods and their still-limited validity has been given in recent years by Cofer & Warren (1962).

Championship and Personality
Of special interest is the problem 'championship and personality'. It is well known that outstanding athletic performances can be accomplished only by a comparatively small number of individuals, and today a champion at international

level is really a product of technique and science applied to a specifically gifted person with a highly developed sense of concentration and exceptional adaptability to stressful effort. The question arises as to what are the characteristic personality features in champions? They can hardly originate from mere desire for muscle building. Their foundation, in my opinion, lies in certain innate mental attitudes, which, if developed by adequate athletic activity, can reach such outstanding high levels of skill as to enable the individual to become the leading personality in a particular field of sport. A strong desire for self-expression can be regarded as a basic feature, associated with a high degree of neuro-muscular co-ordination and self-discipline. Here lies a clear analogy to the outstanding artistic performances in the Arts such as music, sculpture or painting. Only a few studies have been undertaken to analyze the characteristics of champions in sport by experimental psychological tests. Johnson, Hutton & Johnson (1964), in an effort to evaluate the personalities of twelve American champion-class athletes, found as distinguishing characteristics a high level of intellectual ambition, marked self-assurance and absence of inhibition, rendering them capable of powerful emotion and extreme agressiveness. However, as the authors themselves pointed out, the results obtained in this particular group of champions do not justify generalization. It would certainly be of interest to conduct an international study of champions in various sports, in the light of Maslow's concept of self-actualization (1949, 1954), to discover the primary motivation for taking up sport—ie. the mere pleasure of sport, a biological urge, love, or other motives of self-expression.

Sport and Training

Training in sport, defined as "education to efficiency through exercises", has, in the course of years, developed into an important branch of applied physiology. Modern training is a composite of:

(a) interval training, for runners as well as swimmers, with its four variables: length of fast intervals, number of fast intervals, speed of intervals, and length of recovery intervals; (b) Fartlek training: a Swedish expression for speed play; (c) weight training; (d) circuit training, which aims at all-round fitness.

It employs various physiological tests to assess the athlete's physical condition. However, it is a fundamental mistake to believe that the adaptation of man to the stressful efforts of training or the efficiency and precision of the specific functions of sport can be explained merely in terms of quantitative measurements by physiological techniques, such as spiro-ergometry to determine vital capacity and oxygen consumption, by electro-cardiography, telemetry and plethysmography to determine cardiovascular efficiency, by dynamometry and weight-training apparatus or by strength-duration graphs and electromyography to define the extent and intensity of neuromuscular function. It must be remembered that optimal performance-patterns may be subject to great variations, as they depend primarily on the initial posture which the individual type of sport demands. Most of the sports of the able-bodied, in particular field events, fencing, weight-lifting and ball games, are carried out from a standing posture. However, with wheelchair athletes (spinal paraplegics or high double-amputees) the optimum of the performances, for instance in javelin throwing, shot put, club throwing, discus, basketball, weight-lifting, is fundamentally changed because these sports are carried out from a sitting or, as in the case of weight-lifting, a supine position. The efficiency of motion and strength in these athletics depends entirely on the arm, shoulder and trunk muscles. This point will be discussed further in later chapters, but it is mentioned here because it has opened a new field of physiological research and may also be of importance in the training of physical instructors and coaches. Having regard to the continuous development in recent years of wheelchair sports for the physically handicapped, the training of instructors in certain sports and games in a sitting and lying position will undoubtedly widen their knowledge of neuro-muscular function and their understanding of the body and its potential for adaptation.

However, trainers in sport should never lose sight of the psychological state of the trainee and of the fact that the human body is not an automated machine, but that physical performance is a medium of self-expression—a creative outlet which helps to develop personality and character, thus contributing to human development. In training, one is engaged in the first place in self-struggle, with a desire to promote the best abilities and talents one is able to develop in oneself. In this struggle, by obeying the rules of sport, moral qualities, such as self-confidence, initiative, courage, endurance, self-discipline and fairness, as well as team spirit, comradeship and friendship, are developed. These are the virtues which distinguish the real sportsman from a man whose motivation is simply to practise physical exercises for health reasons. But training in sport is also a contest against an opponent, which above all compels courtesy and must be a contest without hate, for sport is not warfare. Naturally, training for sports competitions will encourage the display of the whole of one's energy and the inflexible will to set up higher standards and new records, to win and also to do one's best for the organization and, indeed, the country one represents, but it is also an education in accepting a final decision with grace and without conceit or despondency.

2

Sport and the Physically Handicapped

The Physically Handicapped and the World Around Him

In order to understand the beneficial effects of sport on the severely disabled it is worth while to examine the disabled person's position in the world around him.

(a) Attitude of Society towards the Disabled

It is an undeniable fact that, for thousands of years, the attitude of society towards the severely physically disabled was basically negative, and these unfortunate people were looked upon by the community as outside the accepted norm and as outcasts of society. Many were hidden by their relatives from the eyes of the community as if they would bring shame on the family. The two world wars with their millions of disabled people have certainly changed this attitude, but it is only in comparatively recent times that public opinion generally has recognized the advantage to the community, as well as to the disabled themselves, of making the utmost use of such people and fitting them into suitable places of employment. In particular, the introduction of the modern concepts of rehabilitation after the Second World War has resulted in a positive approach and attitude towards the severely disabled, who are now increasingly accepted as part of the community. The State itself now plays its part in making it a conscious aim of public policy to train the disabled for employment and, through its agencies, to get them jobs on the one hand and include them in recreational and sporting activities on the other. In this respect, the Disabled Persons Employment Act, 1944, and the Chronically Sick and Disabled Persons Employment Act, 1971, in Great Britain have been charters of humanity in improving the attitude of society towards their disabled fellow men. However, there is still room for improvement to enlighten society as a whole that the physically disabled person does not want sympathy or pity but empathy, which is the ability to project one's own personality into that of the physically handicapped, thus acquiring true understanding and full comprehension.

(b) The Attitude of the Disabled towards the Community

It must be remembered that any severe injury or disease resulting in severe disability, such as blindness, deafness, loss of limbs and partial or complete paralysis due to affliction of the nervous system, upsets to a greater or lesser degree the precision, economy and course of the normal movement patterns of the body. The abnormal patterns are characterized by paralysis, weakness, spasticity, stiffness, changes of speech and dysco-ordination. The realization and sudden awareness of the changed body-image resulting from these abnormal patterns of movement is often the cause of a psychological tension between the severely disabled person and his surrounding world, which makes social contact with his able-bodied fellow men difficult and sometimes even impossible. If he is regarded as out of the ordinary by society and continually confronted with embarrassed countenances and staring eyes, a disabled person's attitude to himself may deteriorate into an inferiority complex characterized by shyness, anxiety and loss of self-confidence and personal dignity, and resulting in self-pity, self-isolation and antisocial attitudes.

All these adverse psychological reactions apply to disabled people with otherwise normal intellectual faculties. However, one has to consider also those severely disabled people with congenital or acquired mental disorders, such as children with cerebral palsy (wrongly called 'spastics'), or people of any age who have sustained cerebral injuries resulting in partial paralysis. These disabled individuals need special consideration as special groups for sporting activities, as their aptitude and concentration are diminished; assigning them to the various sports activities is more difficult, requiring specialized medical and psychological assessment. In sport, to mix physically disabled people of normal intellectual and mental capacity with the physically disabled who are mentally retarded or who suffer from other mental and intellectual disorders is as fundamentally wrong as it is to mix able-bodied sportsmen of normal mental ability with those having intellectual or other mental disorders. However, the beneficial effect of sport on the well-being of mentally affected people in promoting interest, concentration and relaxation is in no doubt. Certain psychiatric in-patients of a nearby mental hospital in Aylesbury come three times a week with their nursing attendants to the Stoke Mandeville Sports Stadium for the Paralysed and other Disabled for swimming sessions, which have been a valuable therapeutic factor in their treatment.

The Significance and Aims of Sport for the Disabled

It is not difficult to understand from all this why sport is of even greater significance for the well-being of the severely disabled than it is for the able-bodied. In the following chapter, the aims of sport for the severely disabled as a result of spinal cord injuries will be discussed, but it may be stressed that what is said of these patients can be applied to any other form of severe disability.

Broadly speaking, the aims of sport embody the same principles for the disabled as they do for the able-bodied; in addition, however, sport is of immense therapeutic value and plays an essential part in the physical, psychological and social rehabilitation of the disabled. The aims of sport for the disabled can be summarised as follows:

(a) Sport as a Curative Factor

For the disabled, sport represents the most natural form of remedial exercise and can be successfully employed to complement the conventional methods of physical therapy. It is invaluable in restoring the disabled person's physical fitness, ie. his strength, co-ordination, speed, and endurance. In the contest with himself to improve his performance, the physically handicapped person learns to overcome fatigue, a predominant symptom in the early stages of physical rehabilitation, especially following fractures, amputations and paralysis; the initial cause of the handicap is of little importance.

(b) The Recreational and Psychological Value of Sport

However, sport for the disabled has a deeper meaning than being merely a form of physiotherapy. The great advantage of sport over formal remedial exercise lies in its recreational value, which represents an additional motivation for the disabled by restoring that passion for playful activity and the desire to experience joy and pleasure in life, so deeply inherent in any human being. There is no doubt that much of the benefit of sport, as a form of rehabilitation, is lost if the disabled person does not derive pleasure from its recreative value. Thus, recreation becomes an important factor in promoting that psychological equilibrium which enables the disabled to come to terms with his physical defect. For sport counteracts those adverse psychological attitudes already mentioned which follow with monotonous regularity in the wake of any severe physical disablement. The aims of sport are to develop in the disabled activity of mind, self-confidence, self-dignity, self-discipline, competitive spirit and comradeship, mental attitudes which are essential for getting the disabled person out of the ghetto of self-centred isolation. Therefore, the centuries old slogan *Mens sana in corpore sano*, still so deeply ingrained in society, is no longer valid and should be replaced in future by a new slogan: *Mens sana in corpore sano et invalido!*

(c) Sport as a Means of Social Re-integration

The final—and, I may say, the noblest—aim of sport for the disabled person is to help to restore his contact with the world around him; in other words, to facilitate and accelerate his social re-integration or integration. Regular work in occupational therapy departments and workshops is today generally recognized as a valuable method in the treatment of long-term patients with severe physical defects, to counteract bore-

dom in hospital or institutions and to restore activity of mind and self-confidence. The aims of sport for the disabled are not only identical with those of regular occupation but indeed they greatly amplify them.

There are certain sports and games where the disabled are capable of competing with the able-bodied, for instance, archery, archery darts (dartchery), bowling, snooker and table tennis for the paralysed and amputees, as well as swimming for amputees, the blind and the deaf, which create a better understanding between the disabled and the able-bodied and help the disabled in their social reintegration through the medium of sport. There is no doubt that an employer will not hesitate in appropriate circumstances to employ a paralysed man confined to a wheelchair when he realises that this man is an accomplished sportsman.

3

The Development of Sport for the Disabled—Historical Background

Medicine and Sport

At all times, members of the medical profession concerned with the treatment of deformities and other forms of disability have included physical exercise in their treatment, and gymnastics (the word derives from the Greek word *gumnos*, meaning naked) has through the centuries become a household word for remedial exercise. Erasistratos (305–250 B C) and Galen (131–210) among medical authors of ancient times may be mentioned as advocates of gymnastics. Avicenna (ibn Sina, born 980 A D in Persia) followed Galen's teaching that medical gymnastics should include health-improving exercises. Kruger (1962) quoted Avicenna's poem on medicine: "Do not give up hard exercise, do not seek rest too long; preserve a happy medium. Exercise your limbs to help them repel the bad humors by walking and struggling until you succeed in panting..." Another follower of Galen was Maimonides, the famous medieval Jewish physician. In his *Treatise of Hygiene* (1199 A D) he wrote: "Anyone who lives a sedentary life and does not exercise, even if he eats good foods and takes care of himself according to proper medical principles—all his days will be painful ones and his strength shall wane". Laurent Joubert (1529–1583), Professor of Medicine at the University of Montpellier and an advocate of daily exercise, introduced therapeutic gymnastics into the medical course, as he considered doctors to be the only people really capable of prescribing exercises correctly. During the middle ages and the Renaissance, gymnastics were advocated in various countries. Mercuriale (1530–1608) published in 1569 a treatise of six books *De Arte Gymnastica*, and

Nicholas Andry (1658–1742), who introduced the word 'orthopedie', stressed the great therapeutic value of physical exercises and hydrotherapy. In England, one of the early publications on this subject was Francis Fuller's book, *Medicina Gymnastica—a Treatise on the Power of Exercise with respect to the Animal Economy* (1705), which went to no less than nine editions and, following the 6th edition in 1750, was translated into German. In the beginning of the 19th century, John Shaw (1823) emphasized the beneficial effect of exercises for mild forms of scoliosis: "No single method of treatment is so effectual in counteracting or curing slight distortion of the spine as properly regulated exercises". He warned that this therapy should not be carried out by lay people without medical control. In France, it was Charles Gabriel Pravaz (1790–1853), Guillaume Jalade-Lafond (1827) and Jaques Mathieu Delpech (1828) who pioneered the development of medical gymnastics. In Germany, Jakob Heine (1800–1879) and Daniel Moritz Schreber (1808–1861) founded orthopaedic gymnastics, and Schreber's book *Kinesiatrik oder die gymnastische Heilmethode* (1852), later known as *Ärztliche Zimmer-gymnastik* (Medical-room Gymnastics), in particular, became a very popular book for remedial exercise, with no less than 30 editions. Schreber's name also became famous through his propaganda for the setting up of small plots of ground for gardening as pastime and recreational activities within and around towns, today still called Schrebergarten. In 1845, J.A.L. Werner of Germany published a book based on the anatomical and physiological principles of medical gymnastics for persons suffering from deformities, and two years later the Austrian educationalist, Klein (1847), wrote a book *Gymnastik für Blinde*. The founder of Swedish gymnastics, which were widely accepted in the 19th century and the beginning of the 20th century, was Pehr Henrik Ling (1776–1839). The original Ling's technique was modified by Hendrick Killgren and in this form propagated in Great Britain by Edgar Ferdinand Cyriax (1903), but it was partly replaced in the first quarter of the 20th century by Zander's (1879) technique with the aid of special apparatus. In 1909 R.T. McKenzie, Professor of Physical Education and Physical Therapy, published his book *Exercise in Education and Medicine* which was a fundamental work on the modern concept of the physiology of exercise and rehabilitation. In this connection, the monographs of A.V. Hill of London on *Muscular Movement in Man* and *Living Machinery* (1927) and Bainbridge's book *The Physiology of Muscular Exercise* (1931) have greatly advanced our knowledge of the physiological problems of sport.

These examples may suffice to show how much the medical profession has throughout the centuries recognised the great value of physical exercise and has utilized it in the treatment of disabilities. Since the first World War, this interest in remedial exercise has, in general, vastly increased, and medical specialities such as physical medicine and sports medicine have been created, and in 1928 F I M S was established. Since World War II medical and physiological research on physical education and sport has greatly intensified in many countries.

Own Initiative of Disabled in Sporting Activities

Although disabled people have been encouraged by their medical advisers to take up sport, it is true to say that some handicapped individuals have done this on their own initiative, sometimes against medical advice. They were by no means only those who had already been active in sport before they became handicapped but included people who had never before been interested in sporting activities. This group also includes some who were born with physical defects. In this respect, Lord Byron is a good example. Although handicapped by a congenital leg deformity, he took up rowing and swimming and excelled himself in boxing as a boy and in later life. Diem (1950) published details of Lord Byron's sporting activities. Other examples from the last century are two one-leg amputees, who, each having been provided with a wooden leg, competed with each other in a walking race during a sports festival at Newmarket Heath in England, to the enthusiasm of the spectators (*Athletics*, London, 1880).

With the increasing popularity during the last 30 years of sport in general on the one hand, and the development of sports medicine on the other, it has become more widely recognized that even a major physical defect may not necessarily be an hindrance to high-class performance in sport, provided the disabled person has succeeded, by systematic and intensive training, to mobilise and utilise his remaining abilities and thus compensate for his physical handicap. There are several reports in the literature about soldiers and sportsmen with congenital or acquired heart disease and aortic regurgitation (Parrisius, 1924; Dietlen, 1926; Warfield, 1934; Parade 1936; Jokl & Suzman, 1940). The most interesting cases are those of Parrisius, describing a German ski champion with the symptoms of aortic regurgitation, and of Jokl & Suzman describing a marathon runner, who at the age of 9 had contracted a severe illness which resulted in a valvular disease of the heart with systolic and diastolic murmurs, indicating mitral stenosis and aortic regurgitation. In spite of this physical defect, he took up systematic athletic training and became an outstanding marathon runner in South Africa, winning in 1934 the South African marathon elimination race for the British Empire Games. He further took up training in squash rackets, in which sport he also became prominent. Another interesting case of champion class reported by Jokl in 1957 is the American champion and world record holder in hammer throwing, Harold V. Connolly, who suffered a left-sided arm plexus paralysis of combined Erb-Duchenne and Klumpke-Dejerine type at birth, resulting in paralysis of the finger flexors and small muscles of the fingers of the left hand. The Hungarian Karoly Tacaczs, one of the outstanding pistol marksmen, who lost his right arm in 1938 following an accident, transferred his skill by intensive training to his left arm which he had never used previously. He became Olympic champion in this sport in London 1948 and Helsinki in 1952 (Frucht, 1960). One of my former paraplegic patients, Mrs. Margaret Harriman who became an outstanding archer and who lives in South Africa, was chosen to represent that country in a championship competition of able-bodied archers held some years ago in Norway and came 8th out of 48 competitors.

If a disabled person had already mastered a certain sport prior to his disability, he may even utilize this particular sport in addition to conventional methods of physiotherapy to conquer his disability. He may even regain his former skill to such an extent as to be able to compete in high-class competitions with both other disabled and with able-bodied competitors. Amputees have adapted themselves with striking ability to sports in which they were skilled prior to their injury. I have attended swimming contests of amputees in various countries and have always been deeply impressed by the skill and prowess of double amputees, especially those with high, above-knee amputations, in distance competitions, and by the diving performances from the highest spring-board of one-leg or one-arm amputees. In Austria, Finland, France and Germany, leg and arm-amputees, who before their injuries were expert skiers, have regained their skill after amputation. A former Austrian skiing teacher, who lost both legs below the knee in the Second World War, was able to resume his occupation as a ski teacher after regaining his skill. The same applies to the sport of golf. Skilled golfers have taken up the game again after amputation and in this connection,

one of the outstanding officers of the Royal Air Force in the Second World War, Group Captain Douglas Bader may be mentioned. He had both legs amputated before the war following an air crash (one above the knee, the other below the knee). He flew during the war as a most successful commander and still plays a strenuous game of golf off a handicap of six, and engages in other sports (see later).

Lis Hartel, the well-known Danish equestrienne, is an outstanding example of the conquest of severe paralysis as a result of affliction of the spinal cord acquired at a later time in life. She started riding at the age of eight and became an expert horsewoman, especially in dressage. In 1944, at the age of 23, while expecting her second child, she was stricken with severe poliomyelitis during the epidemics in Denmark, which left her partially paralysed for life in both lower limbs. It is interesting and moving to read Lis Hartel's own account of her gradual recovery by constant exercises, published in Sir Ian Fraser's (later Lord Fraser of Lonsdale) book *Conquest of Disability*. Crawling first with her little daughter on the floor, she eventually recovered to such a degree that she decided to the amazement of her family and friends, to try riding again. This is how she described her first attempt: "The first sensation was indescribable, and a profound joy and sense of gratitude seized me. I felt that one of my aims had been achieved and that the next was waving to me in the distance. I was so sore and tired after that first ride that I had to go to bed again, and about a fortnight went by before I could make my next attempt". She continued her riding exercises relentlessly and systematically, and by doing this discovered what a useful exercise riding could be for a great number of polio victims. She explains the over-all training effect of riding on the muscular system, as compared with exercises of conventional mechanical devices, as follows: "A horse is not a machine or piece of gymnastic apparatus. Although its movements are regular, they are nevertheless subject to variations, and a diversity of situa-

tions can arise which force the rider uncons-
ciously to use or attempt to use some groups of
muscles or other, and at the same time every
muscle and sinew in his body is 'massaged' or
worked on in some way." At the Olympic
Games in Helsinki in 1952, eight years after the
onset of her paralysis, she came second in the
most difficult dressage competition and won a
silver medal.

Blind people take interest in road walking to
restore their balance and orientation in space.
At St. Dunstan's, road-walking contests have
been held throughout the years for war-blinded
ex-servicemen. One of them, Tommy Gaygan,
mentioned by Basil Curtis in Sir Ian Fraser's
book *Conquest of Disability*, who was blinded
and in addition lost both hands during the desert
battles of the 8th Army in the Second World
War, became interested in this contest and in due
course beat most of his blind comrades in their
races around Regent's Park in London. For some
time, he was the St. Dunstan's champion, and at
his best he was able to cover nearly seven miles
in an hour, which, as Curtis rightly remarks, is
"some going, whether you are blind or not".

Development of Sports Organisations for the Disabled

In spite of these examples of outstanding
achievements in sport by severely disabled individuals, organised competitive sport amongst
larger groups of handicapped people is a rela-
tively new development. Although sports organisation for the deaf were formed in various countries before the first world war—in Germany the
first sports club for the deaf was started in
Berlin in 1888—increasing interest in sport,
especially amongst amputees and the blind was
aroused during and after the first world war.
However, the initial enthusiasm of the disabled
themselves did not last in Germany, in spite of
the efforts of physicians and surgeons such as
Mallwitz, Biesalsky, Kohlrausch, Diem, Schede,
and Würtz, and only small groups of disabled,
mainly amputees, continued sporting activities
in various countries.

In England, the Disabled Drivers' Motor
Club, which has over 900 members and is now
recognized by the Government as the representative organisation of disabled motorists, was
founded in 1922. This Club organises frequent
rallies and competitive events, and has in recent
years held its Annual meeting at the sportsground of Stoke Mandeville Hospital, Aylesbury, with competitions of skill for amputees,
paralysed and other disabled people. Some of
the tests are extremely difficult and one can only
wish that many able-bodied motorists could
achieve the same degree of skill. Amongst the
competitors has been a polio victim with complete paralysis of both arms who has learned to
drive a specially adapted car with his feet. He
also paints with his feet.

The British Society of One-Armed Golfers is
another pre-war sports organisation; it was
founded in 1932 in the offices of A. Pollock, a
Glasgow solicitor, and holds its annual championships on leading courses throughout the
country. A later development was the National
Golf Amputee Association of America, for both
arm and leg amputees. The British Society of
One-Armed Golfers has about 90 members of
varying ages and occupations; some of their disabilities are congenital, some arise from injuries
from both World Wars, and others are the result
of industrial and other accidents. All members
must play every stroke with one arm, and no aid
from the stump of the amputated arm or from
an artificial appliance is allowed. While most
players play off a handicap between 15 and
24, the more efficient play off a club handicap
of between 8 and 14. According to R.D.
Marshall, President of the British Society, the
best British one-armed player is the St. Andrews'
golfer R.P. Reid, who today plays off a handicap
of 4.

Sport and Rehabilitation during and after World War II

The Second World War, with its large numbers
of disabled, provided a new and great incentive
for reviving the idea of sport as an aid to the

treatment and rehabilitation of war disabled, and this was practised particularly in Great Britain, U.S.A. and Germany. In England, within a few months of the outbreak of the war, the late Sir Reginald Watson Jones, the orthopaedic surgeon, then civilian consultant to the Royal Air Force, established a complete rehabilitation service for orthopaedic injuries in the R.A.F., in which the late Group Captain O'Malley took a leading part. Amongst the methods of remedial exercises employed in the R.A.F. Rehabilitation Units were periods of games, such as cricket and tug-of-war, which proved highly successful from both physical and psychological points of view.

In Germany, it was Mallwitz in particular who, from his experience during and after the First World War, promoted gymnastics and sport as part of the rehabilitation of war-injured soldiers in military hospitals such as Berlin-Buch and Hohenlychen, and in 1943 this was officially accepted by the authorities concerned. However, there, as in this country, sporting activities were confined mainly to patients with fractures of the limbs, amputees and the blind.

The Development of Hetero(Multi)-Disabled Sports Organisations

Sport for amputees and the blind has greatly developed since the Second World War and still plays a major part in sport for the disabled in most countries of the European Continent as well as in Canada, India, Indonesia, Israel, Korea, Japan and South Africa. Disabled ex-service-men from World War II, supported and guided by their medical advisers, themselves took the initiative to start sports clubs. In Germany in 1949, for instance, the sports educator Weinmann in co-operation with Dr. Winke organised the first sports competition of war invalids in Göppingen and, in 1950, the first skiing competition for amputees took place in Bavaria under the guidance of the orthopaedic surgeons Lange and Witt. In 1951, *Der Deutsche Versehrtensportverband* (D V S—German Assoc-

iation of Sport for the Physically Handicapped) was founded through the initiative of leading members of the V D K, the German Ex-servicemen's Associations, such as Mallwitz, Bazille, Brinkmann, Lorenzen, Rosslenbroich, Tüffers and others. The sports teacher Hans Lorenzen, of the Sports-Hochschule, Cologne, where its Rector Professor C. Diem created a Chair of Sport for the Disabled, published in 1961 a very comprehensive and well illustrated textbook on Sport for the Disabled (*Lehrbuch des Versehrtensports*) with special emphasis on amputees. The D V S was recognised by the Government of the West German Republic as the governing body of Sport for the disabled of all types, both civilians and ex-servicemen. In 1953 a Sports Sanatorium was opened in Isny with American financial help.

The Fédération Française du Sport pour Handicapées Physiques developed as a hetero-disabled sports organisation also through the initiative of ex-servicemen, especially Berthe and Avronsart from the early fifties, and the Austrian Sports Organisation for the Hetero-Disabled developed under the leadership of Deschka, Reindl, Schindlauer and Dr. Wechselberger, the Finnish under Piirto, Reihaimo, Petrala, the Belgian under Boin, Dr. Houssa and Dr. Tricot, the Yugoslavian under the late Grga Jankes and Branco Golovic, and the Dutch under Westerhoff, Tjebbes and Dr. van der Maas. All these organisations started in the early post-war period and have developed ever since to embrace all forms of hetero-disability. These countries were followed by Canada, Czechoslovakia, East Germany, Israel, Japan, Indonesia, Luxembourg, Norway, Poland, Spain, Sweden and Switzerland.

The British Sports Association for Hetero(Multi)-Disabled (BSAD)

The success of the sports movement for the paralysed has been a great incentive and inspiration to people with other disabilities to take up sport as a pastime and recreation. It seemed worth while therefore to combine the sporting activities of these people, particularly amputees, the blind, and those with cerebral palsy and spinal paralysis, in hetero-disabled sports contests. This led to the foundation, in 1961, of the British Sports Association for the Disabled (B S A D) with headquarters at Stoke Mandeville Sports Stadium which are provided rent free by the B P S S. B S A D has its own administrator, two technical officers, one sports development officer for the regions and a shorthand typist. B S A D has its own constitution and Executive Council of twelve members which is responsible for all the activities of this sports organisation and holds regular meetings during the year. The B S A D has been recognized by the British Government and its Sports Council, as well as by the Central Council of Physical Recreation, as the Governing Body for all types of sport for disabled persons in Great Britain, and, since 1964, has been entitled to Government grants, just as is any sports organization for the able-bodied. In 1972, B S A D, at the request of the Sports Council, divided the whole country into ten Regions, each of which works in close liaison with its local authorities and with the Regional Sports Councils, as well as with B S A D Headquarters. Regional sports competitions are held to select competitors for the National Hetero-Disabled Games at Stoke Mandeville. Since its inception, B S A D has held annual sports festivals in which amputees, the blind and those suffering from cerebral palsy and spinal cord afflictions, including spina bifida, muscular dystrophy and the milder forms of multiple sclerosis take part. In early July these annual multi-disabled games are reserved for youngsters from the age of 8 to 16; in September or October the annual games are held for adults of varying age. The number of participating competitors varies between 300 and 400. The sports competitions include archery, field and track events, including races, relays and slalom, basketball, shinty, volley ball, swimming, table tennis and bowling, and the standards of achievement are steadily increasing from year to year. The number of youngsters competing in these games has increased, in 1975, to more than 500, and steps are being considered to divide the games into two separate age-groups and to increase the number of days allotted to this annual sports festival. B S A D also takes part in international competitions and is a founder member of the International Sports Organisation for the Hetero-Disabled (I S O D).

The International Sports Organisation for Hetero(Multi)-Disabled (I S O D)

In 1960, an International Working Group on Sport for the Disabled was set up under the aegis of the World Veterans Federation (W V F). Unfortunately, this Working Group was beset with difficulties from the beginning, not merely as a result of language difficulties, but mainly due to differences of opinion about the objects to be pursued. It was dissolved in 1964 and replaced by I S O D with a membership of 16 nations, at first under the Patronage of W V F. However, in 1967 I S O D became an independent international sports organisation for the hetero- or multi-disabled, including amputees, the blind and those with cerebral palsy or spinal cord afflictions, but its aim, as a coordinating body, is also to embrace other disabilities in the future. In the same year, headquarters were transferred from Paris, to England, where its administration is accommodated at Stoke Mandeville Stadium. Its first General Secretary was Charles Dunham M B E, General Secretary of the British Limbless Ex-servicemen's Association (B L E S M A) who, unfortunately, had to resign due to ill-health and his post was taken over by Joan Scruton M B E, General Secretary of B P S S. I S O D has its own constitution and praesidium which holds regular meetings, as a rule twice a year. Dr. Adam Bilik (Poland) acts as the Medical Officer and Sepp Reindl (Austria) as Technical Officer. The members of the praesidium are elected by the General Assembly of member nations, but once elected they are independent and not just representatives of their

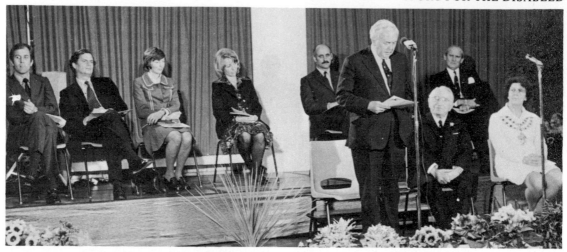

Fig. 1   The British Prime Minister, the Rt. Hon. Harold Wilson, at the opening of
the First World Multi-Disabled Games at Stoke Mandville Sports Stadium in 1974.

own countries. International rules for sports for amputees and the blind have been worked out and amended throughout the years and those for cerebral palsy are in preparation. For the paralysed, the rules of I S M G F have been accepted as obligatory by I S O D. A Sports Calendar has been compiled for national and international multi-disabled games in co-operation with the I S M G F. I S O D has accepted patronage of international hetero-disabled sports meetings in various countries including Austria, Belgium, France, Poland and Spain and in September 1974 the first Hetero-Disabled World Games were organised at the request of I S O D by the B S A D at Stoke Mandeville Sports Stadium for the Paralysed and other Disabled, where 212 competitors (amputees, blind and paralysed) representing 26 countries, and observers from seven other countries, took part. These games, which were officially opened by the Prime Minister of Great Britain, the Rt. Hon. Harold Wilson, (Fig. 1) were a great success, and the standards of performance and, above all, the spirit of sportsmanship were excellent. The games provided a good opportunity to try out in practice the accepted rules for amputees and the blind, and as a result of the experience gained, amendments and alterations have become necessary and have been elaborated and accepted by the Praesidium of I S O D. The new rules will be applied in 1976 at the Olympiad for the Physically Disabled in Toronto which will be held in co-operation between ISOD and ISMGF. Altogether 1700 competitors will take part—1100 paraplegics and tetraplegics and 600 amputees and blind sportsmen.

4

Wheelchair Sports
for Spinal Para- and Tetraplegics

The Old Concept of Spinal Cord Paralysis

It was not until the later stages of the Second World War that sport as a part of medical treatment was introduced by the author in Great Britain to a group of wounded soldiers suffering from one of the most devastating disablements which can beset mankind, spinal paraplegia. Until then, it would have been quite inconceivable to assume that gymnastic activities, let alone competitive sport, could play a part in the treatment of people paralysed from the waist, chest and even higher levels, as a result of injury or disease of the spinal cord. Such people are called paraplegics (when the paralysis affects the lower limbs and trunk) and tetraplegics (when the paralysis also involves the upper limbs). The proper Greek term tetraplegia is often replaced by many specialists, especially in USA and Canada, by the confusing terms quadr*i*plegia, quadr*a*plegia and quadr*u*plegia which should really be abandoned for the sake of uniformity of terminology. Throughout the centuries, up to the time of the Second World War, spinal paraplegics, let alone tetraplegics, were considered by most members of the medical profession, even those who had otherwise accepted and practised the philosophy of rehabilitation of disabled people, as hopeless cripples, with a short duration of life—as a rule no longer than two to three years. The causes of their early deaths were complications resulting from their spinal cord injury which were considered as inevitable, namely general sepsis from bedsores and infection of the paralysed bladder resulting in destruction of the kidneys. The view generally held was that very little or nothing could be done for them and the sooner they died the better for all concerned. Spinal paraplegia, unlike blindness and amputation, did not constitute a social problem to the community at large. Those who survived any length of time were kept in institutions for incurables or at home, a burden to everyone and to themselves. This defeatist attitude on the part of the medical profession was naturally shared by members of the para-medical professions—nurses and physiotherapists—and for the public as a whole paraplegics were the subject of charity or a focus of curiosity.

Spinal Injuries Units were set up during the Second World War in Great Britain, for it was generally agreed that conditions for a systematic study of this complex problem of spinal paraplegia were more favourable in a spinal unit than when the patients lay scattered in general medical or surgical wards or in specialised units such as neuro-surgical or orthopaedic departments with only their restricted facilities for short-term treatments. There were, however, several reasons why the first spinal units did not succeed in changing fundamentally the depressing outlook of these unfortunate victims of the war, the most important being that no one member of the medical and nursing staff devoted more than part of his or her time to the care of spinal injury patients. There was no definite plan or objective for the rehabilitation of even the more fit patients, with consequently no real change in this depressing and most neglected aspect of medicine.

Clinical Sport—A New Approach

In February 1944 at the request of the Government, the author of this book opened the Spinal

Injuries Centre at Stoke Mandeville Hospital in Aylesbury, as one of the medical preparations for the second front. In this centre, the concept of Comprehensive Mangement and Rehabilitation of spinal cord sufferers was introduced; it was a new approach, based on the following principles, namely:

(1) that the complications resulting from a spinal cord injury, such as sepsis from bedsores and infection of the urinary tract, causing suffering and the early death of paraplegics, are by no means as inevitable as was commonly thought, but can be controlled and even avoided altogether, provided all aspects of immediate, early and long-term care are understood.

(2) that, by mobilising and developing the dormant forces of natural repair, as well as those of re-adjustment and compensatory function of the neuro-muscular system of the paralysed, not only can their life-expectation be prolonged but their return to a new life of independence, usefulness and dignity can be achieved.

(3) to accomplish this, for the first time in the medical management of these patients the hitherto customary fragmentation of treatment carried out in different surgical and medical specialties was replaced by comprehensive management of all aspects of the complex problem of spinal cord injury dealt with by a specialised staff from the day of injury and throughout all stages of hospital treatment and social rehabilitation. The work of the whole team was directed and co-ordinated by an experienced specialist—in the author's case a surgical neurologist—who was prepared to give up part of his own specialty in order to devote his full time to the work in this multi-disciplinary speciality of medicine and surgery, which demanded meticulous attention to detail and, by no means least, involved co-ordinating the sometimes conflicting interests of the visiting medical and surgical specialists concerned with the special problems of the treatment of paraplegics and tetraplegics.

It was obvious that radical changes in the medical and psychological approach to the problem of paraplegia as a whole and the introduction of new methods of physiotherapy in particular, were imperative. Certain traditional methods of treatment were rejected and replaced by new, sometimes unorthodox procedures. Among the methods of the new approach to the management of paraplegica, sport proved a fundamentally new concept and has ever since played a paramount part in the physical, psychological and social rehabilitation of these severely physically handicapped people Guttmann 1945–1975).

It was the consideration of the over-all training effect of sport on the neuro-muscular system and because it seemed the most natural form of recreation to prevent boredom in hospital which, in 1944 following successful experiments with punchball exercises (Fig. 2), darts, rope-climbing (Fig. 3), skittles and snooker, led me to introduce wheelchair polo as the first competitive team sport for paraplegics, to which very soon badminton and wheelchair basketball were added. The idea of competitive team sport for paraplegics was born on an afternoon in the autumn of 1944, when I tried to move about in a wheelchair and, using the curved handle of a walking stick as a mallet, hit a ball and chase after it, at the same time trying to prevent my opponent in a wheelchair—the physical instructor of the hospital, the late Mr. T.S. Hill—from counteracting my movements. However clumsy our performance may have been, it taught me two things:

(1) that wheelchair polo, as I had already termed it in my mind, was possible as a competitive team sport for paraplegics.

(2) judging from my own and my opponent's difficulty in manoeuvring the chair and keeping our legs still in position, a sport was about to be created in which the

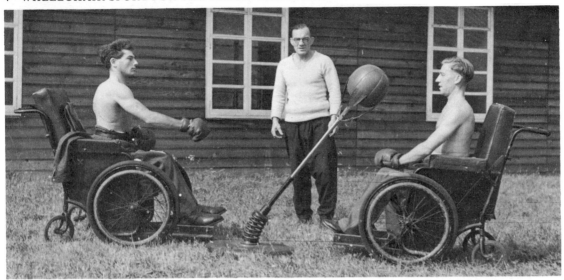

paraplegic was clearly less handicapped than the able-bodied. For, having regard to the diversity of movements necessary in contest with an opponent, it is extremely difficult for the able-bodied person to keep his feet still in the tray or on the foot rest of the chair, whilst manoeuvring it and pushing a disc or weighted ball with a mallet and one is liable to fall out of one's chair. Actually, in due course, any wheelchair team of able-bodied-players was hopelessly beaten by the paraplegic polo-teams.

At the beginning of 1945, however, wheelchair polo was replaced by wheelchair basketball as a more suitable team game, which later became the most popular and fascinating team sport of the paralysed.

Archery and table tennis were also introduced as new sports.

These experiments were the beginning of a systematic development of competitive sport for the paralysed as an essential part of their medical rehabilitation and social re-integration in the community of a country like Great Britain where sport in one form or another plays such

Fig. 2   Punchball exercises during hospital treatment.

Fig. 3   Rope-climbing exercises by a man with a complete paraplegia below T 6.

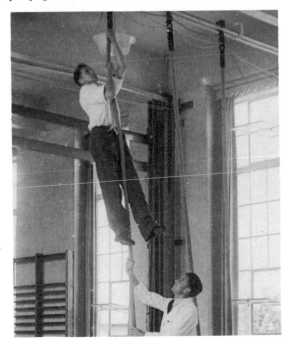

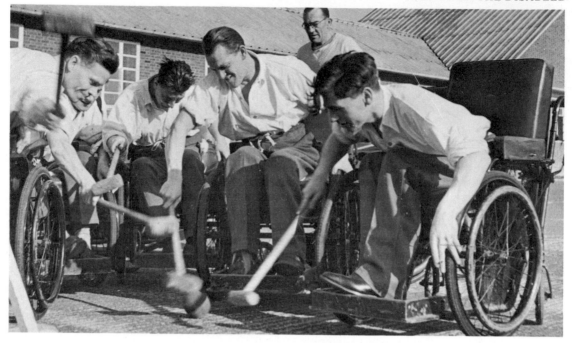

Fig. 4   1945—a beginning! The first wheelchair team sport—polo.

an essential part in the life of so many people. This idea has since spread all over the world.

Development of the Stoke Mandeville Games as the Olympics of the Paralysed

The success of sport as remedial exercise and clinical treatment provided the incentive to start a sports movement for the paralysed. It was on the 28th July 1948 that the Stoke Mandeville Games for the Paralysed were founded as an annual sports festival, with only 16 British ex-members of the Armed Forces (14 men and 2 women) as competitors. This competition took place on the same day that the Olympic Games were opened in London. Small as it was, it was a demonstration to the public that competitive sport is not the prerogative of the able-bodied but that the severely disabled, even those with a disablement of such magnitude as spinal paraplegia, can become sportsmen and women in their own right. The Games were an immediate

success and an inspiration to spinal cord sufferers in other parts of the country. As each annual sports day came round, the number of competitors and sports events increased. In the early years the games were opened with club-swinging demonstrations to musical accompaniment, given by patients of the Spinal Unit in the early stages of rehabilitation (Fig. 5). At the prize-giving ceremony in 1949, I was somewhat carried away by the success of the Games that year, and, looking into the future, expressed the hope that the time might come when this event "would be truly international and the Stoke Mandeville Games would achieve world fame as the disabled men and women's equivalent of the Olympic Games" (*The Cord*, 1949, **3,** 24). That dream became reality in 1952, when the Games became international by the participation of a team of Dutch paralysed ex-servicemen. Altogether 58 countries have so far been represented at these Games, which in itself shows the development of spinal paraplegia as a world-

Fig. 5 Indian club-swinging demonstration at Stoke Mandeville Hospital

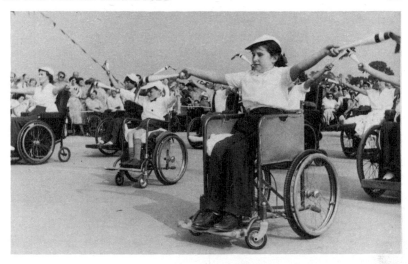

wide problem.

An International Stoke Mandeville Games Committee was formed, and it was decided that these Games should take place at the end of July each year in memory of their foundation in the sports ground of Stoke Mandeville Hospital, with the exception of every fourth year, when they should be held in the Country where the Olympic Games take place, provided adequate arrangements could be made. Moreover, the International Stoke Mandeville Games differ from the Olympics and other international sports events of the able-bodied, as they are not confined only to champions but are open also to moderately-advanced wheelchair athletes.

The first International Stoke Mandeville Games outside Stoke Mandeville were held in the Olympic year 1960 in Rome, when 400 paralysed sportsmen and women representing 23 countries joined in the competitions held at the

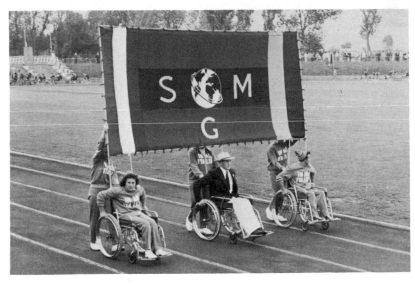

Fig. 6 The Stoke Mandeville Games banner, carried by a British and two Italian competitors, entering the Stadium in Rome at the 1960 Olympic Games of the Paralysed.

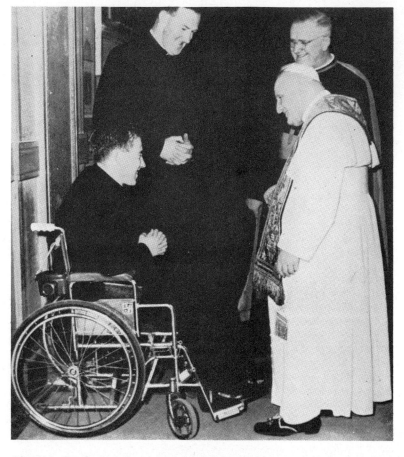

Fig. 7   Pope John XXIII giving a personal audience to Father Leo Close.

Olympic Stadium following the Olympic Games and under Olympic Games conditions (Fig. 6). The Games were opened by Donna Carla Gronchi, wife of the President of the Italian Republic, and they aroused great interest amongst the public. At the end of the Games the late Pope John XXIII gave a special audience in the Vatican City to all competitors and their 300 escorts. The effect the Games made on the public could not have been better expressed than by Pope John who said "You are the living demonstration of the marvels of the virtue of energy. You have given a great example, which we would like to emphasize, because it can be a lead to all: you have shown what an energetic soul can achieve, in spite of apparently insur-

mountable obstacles imposed by the body." Fig. 7 shows the late Pope John XXIII giving a private audience to Father Leo Close from Dublin, a former paraplegic patient at the National Spinal Injuries Centre, Stoke Mandeville, following fracture of the spine, and a competitor at the Rome Games. He was ordained by special permission of Pope John after passing his exam and became the first Catholic priest 'on wheels'. He has been for many years Director of Education in Dunedin, New Zealand and still takes part in national and international games of the paralysed.

The second occasion was in Tokyo in November 1964, where 370 wheelchair athletes from 23 nations competed in the magnificent new

Fig. 8   Opening of the 1964 Olympics of the Paralysed in Tokyo by T.I.H. The Crown Prince and Crown Princess of Japan.

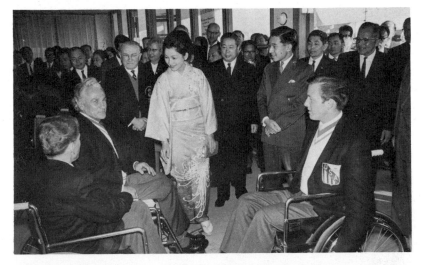

Fig. 9   Scene at the closing ceremony of the Tokyo Games.

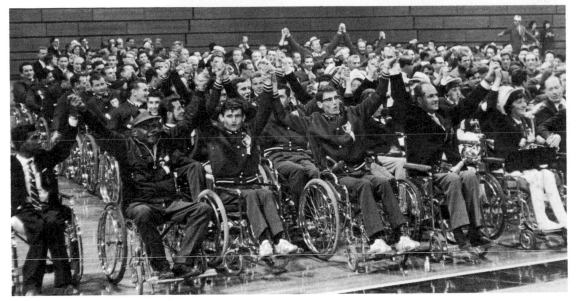

Olympic Stadium immediately after the Olympic Games. The Games were opened by T.I.H. The Crown Prince and his wife Princess Mishiko, and members of the Imperial Family, including The Empress, attended the Games during the week (Figs. 8 & 9). The public took a great interest in these Games, as evidenced by the attendance of more than 100,000 spectators.

The Tokyo Games were outstanding in demonstrating the effect of sport of the disabled on society as a whole. The Japanese Government, having realised the capabilities of men and women in a wheelchair in the field of sport, and recognising the immense value of sport in the social rehabilitation of the severely disabled, within six months set up a factory for paraplegic

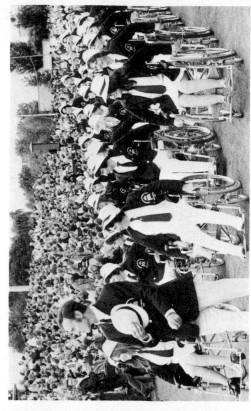

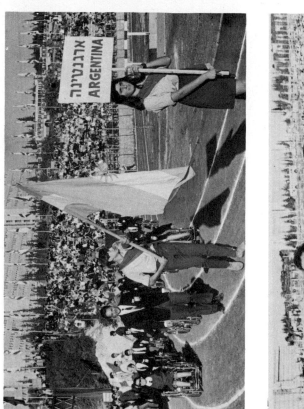

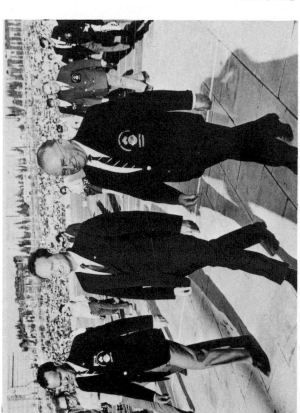

Fig. 10 Opening ceremony, 1968 Olympics of the Paralysed at the University Stadium, Jerusalem. *Above, left:* Wheelpast of Nations; *right:* The British team in the Wheelpast of Nations. *Left:* Arrival of Mr Ygal Allon, Deputy Prime Minister of Israel, with Mr Arieh Fink, Chairman of the Israeli Stoke Mandeville Games Committee, and Sir Ludwig Guttmann.

Fig. 11   1972 Olympics of
the Paralysed, Heidelberg.
Upper: Dr. Heinemann,
President of the German
Federal Republic, greeting the
representative of Israel on the
right of whom is the repre-
sentative of the German team.
Lower: Presentation of the
Olympic flag to the President
of the Games by Professor V.
Praeslack, Chairman of the
Organising Committee at
the final ceremony of the
Games.

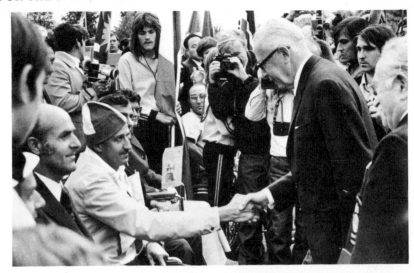

and other severely disabled workers. There are
at present four such factories in Japan, called
Sun Industries, of which Dr. Nakamura, an
orthopaedic surgeon and former graduate of the
Stoke Mandeville Spinal Centre, is in charge.

In 1968 it was not possible, as planned, to
hold the Games in Mexico in connection with
the Olympic Games, due to difficulties in organisation on the part of the Mexican authorities.
They were held instead at Ramat Gan, near Tel
Aviv in Israel, with 750 competitors and 350
escorts representing 29 countries. The Games
were opened in the large University Stadium in
Jerusalem (Fig. 10) by Mr. Ygal Allon the Deputy
Prime Minister, who deputized for the Prime
Minister who was sick. In his address, Mr.
Allon pointed out: "We would have been very
happy to welcome paralyzed sportsmen from
the Arabic countries". The President of the
State, Mr. Shazar, received representatives of all
nations at his residence. The public followed the
Games enthusiastically and a crowd of 25,000
attended the Opening Ceremony at the University Sports Stadium in Jerusalem and the daily
sports events in Ramat Gan were attended by
many spectators. The final basketball match between the Israeli and American teams at Ramat

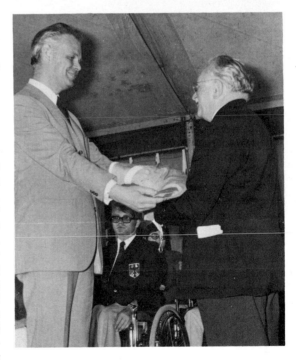

Gan was attended by about 5000 people and a
large crowd who could not get into the Stadium
because of lack of space had to be turned back

by mounted police. General Dayan, who was the guest of honour, presented the trophies to the winning Israeli team.

In the Olympic year of 1972, the Games were held from the 2nd to 10th August in Heidelberg, Germany, in the newly built Sports Stadium, where 1000 paralysed athletes representing 44 countries took part. The University and the City of Heidelberg opened their doors and hearts to enable the 21st International Stoke Mandeville Games to be held in that famous city, under the aegis of the D V S (Deutscher Versehrten Sportsverband) but organised by national and local committees under the chairmanship of Professor V. Paeslack, Director of the Spinal Injuries Centre of the Orthopaedic University Clinic in Heidelberg and his organising secretary Mr. Walter Weiss, Director of the Berufsförderungs Institute, Wilbad. The 1000 competitors and their 400 escorts were accommodated in the Berufsförderungswerk in Heidelberg (the Industrial Rehabilitation Centre), the Director of which, Mr. W. Boll, put all the magnificent facilities of this Centre at our disposal. The Games were opened by Dr. Gustav Heineman, the President of the Federal Republic of Germany (Fig. 11). In his address, the President said: "It is an honour for The Federal Republic of Germany to be the host of these Games. At the same time, it is a great responsiblity to fulfil the very important socio-political duty reaching beyond these games, namely the integration of disabled persons in all walks of life. The disabled person not only participates in a normal profession, but also functions as a fully valid member of a community. The International Stoke Mandeville Games are a proof of this. It was, therefore, with great pleasure that I accepted the patronage of the games."

The development of the Stoke Mandeville Games since their inception in 1948 can be seen in Table 1.

The fact that it was not possible to hold the Olympiad for the Paralysed in Mexico or Munich in connection with the Olympic Games raises an important point of principle which will be discussed further in the chapter on sports facilities for the disabled.

TABLE 1

YEAR	PLACE	NO. OF COMPETITORS
1948	SM	16
1949	SM	60
1950	SM	110
1951	SM	126
1952	SM(I)	130
1953	SM	200
1954	SM	250
1955	SM	280
1956	SM	300
1957	SM	360
1958	SM	350
1959	SM	360
1960	ROME (O)	400
1961	SM	240
1962	SM	320
1963	SM	363
1964	TOKYO (O)	390
1965	SM	390
1966	SM	360
1967	SM	370
1968	TEL-AVIV (O)	750
1969	SM	450
1970	SM	415
1971	SM	430
1972	HEIDELBERG (O)	1000
1973	SM	550
1974	SM	560
1975	SM	630

SM = Stoke mandeville
I = International for the first time
O = Olympic Year

Development of Wheelchair Sport in other Countries

Many countries have followed our example and have adopted wheelchair sport for the spinal paralysed.

Europe

Austria, Belgium, Czechoslovakia, Denmark, Finland, France, Germany (both the Federal Republic and East Germany), Ireland, Italy, Holland, Malta, Norway, Poland, Portugal, Spain, Sweden and Yugoslavia have developed sport for paraplegics and most of them have taken part in the annual I S M G regularly for many years, Holland, as mentioned before, having been the co-founder of the Games in 1952.

North America

The USA has pioneered wheelchair sport since 1946/47 under the leadership of Ben Lipton and his Committee, and has taken part regularly in the I S M G. While paraplegics in USA at first trained and practised basketball almost exclusively and achieved outstanding skill, they later adopted most of the other sports practised during the Stoke Mandeville Games.

Canada was rather late in developing wheelchair sport, but in recent years, especially after our Olympics in Israel and Germany, Canada has made great strides in this respect under the leadership of Dr. R. Jackson, Dr. Grogono and Dick Loiselle.

South America

Argentina. Dr. Cibeira and Hector Ramirez have organised sports for the paralysed in Argentina, who have taken part regularly in the annual I S M G.

Brazil. In recent years this country also has developed wheelchair sport and has taken part in the I S M G, as have Chile, Mexico and Peru.

Colombia. In recent years, this country has also developed sport amongst the paralysed and has already taken part on two occasions. Particular interest was aroused in this country after an International Congress of Physiotherapy in 1970.

West Indies. In this part of the world, Jamaica is outstanding in the development of sport for the paralysed, under the leadership of Sammy Henriques and Professor John Golding. This country has taken part in the I S M G, the Pan-American Games and the Commonwealth Paraplegic Games.

Middle East Countries

Israel was the first Middle-Eastern country to participate and has for many years taken part regularly in the annual I S M G. In the Spewack Centre at Ramat Gan, Gershon Huberman and his co-workers have done pioneer work in training the paralysed. A S M G Committee was founded in Israel under the Chairmanship of Arieh Fink, who is responsible for the development and organisation of wheelchair sport.

Egypt. In recent years, Egypt also developed wheelchair sport under the leadership of Admiral Latif, and has taken part in our annual Games, with increasing numbers of competitors.

Africa

The countries of the African continent which have developed sport for paraplegics include Ethiopia and Kenya, where John Britton from England founded the first Spinal Unit in Nairobi. Furthermore, both South Africa and Rhodesia have developed sport for the paralysed and have taken part in the I S M G since 1962, and the South African Government has recently agreed to send to the I S M G—for the first time—a mixed racial team which has been selected on merit only and not, as in previous years, on racial partition. This is really the first breakthrough in the apartheid problem, achieved by the sports movement of the paralysed. During my recent visit to South Africa to attend a congress on rehabilitation held in Cape Town, I witnessed three basketball matches, between mixed coloured and white competitors.

Sudan has been represented since 1974 and Uganda on two occasions.

South Pacific

Australia was the first country in this area to develop sport for the disabled, organised by Dr George Bedbrook in Perth who brought the first Australian team to Stoke Mandeville in 1957.

New Zealand also has formed a sports organisation and taken part in our Olympics; moreover, the latest Commonwealth Paraplegic Games were held in Dunedin, New Zealand.

Far East

Here Japan pioneered sport for paraplegics under the leadership of Mr. Kasai and Dr. Nakamura, and in 1964 Olympics for the Paralysed were held in Tokyo, which were particularly important from the point of social reintegration of the paralysed into the community.

Other Far Eastern countries that have taken part in our Games for several years are Hong Kong, India, Malaysia, Korea and the Philippines.

British Commonwealth Paraplegic Games

At the instigation of Dr. George Bedbrook, the first British Commonwealth Paraplegic Games were held in 1962 at Perth, Australia, the second in 1966 in Jamaica, the third in 1970 at Edinburgh, Scotland and the fourth at Dunedin, New Zealand. These Games were, of course, on a smaller scale than the I S M G. At the last British Commonwealth Paraplegic Games it was recommended to the I S M G F that the time had come to set up World Zone Games in which perhaps, members of the British Commonwealth countries could give a lead, and this was accepted.

World Zone Games for the Paralysed

The steadily increasing interest by the paralysed in sporting activities has led to the formation of the following World Zone Games as offshoots of the Stoke Mandeville Games.

European Zone

European Games have been held since 1957 in Austria, Belgium, France, Germany, Holland, Italy, Poland and Sweden.

Pan American Zone

Pan-American Games were held for the first time in 1967 at Winnipeg, Canada, for the second at Buenos Aires, in 1969, the third at Kingston, Jamaica in 1971, the fourth in Chile in 1973 and the fifth in Mexico in 1975.

Far Eastern and South Pacific Zone (FESPIC Games)

The first Games of this last area were held in June 1975 at Oita, South Japan, organised by Dr. Nakamura and Mr. Kasai, and were opened by The Crown Prince and Crown Princess of Japan. In addition to countries such as Australia, Hong Kong, India, Japan, Korea and New Zealand, Bangladesh, Burma, Indonesia, Malaysia, Pakistan, Philippines, Sri Lanka, Thailand and even Papua, New Guinea took part. These Games were held under the aegis of both I S M G F and I S O D and were a great success. It may be mentioned that the organising country, Japan, even paid the air fares of the representatives of those countries who could not afford it.

Who would have thought, when the Stoke Mandeville Games started 28 years ago with 16 people, that one day paraplegics and even tetraplegics from all parts of the world would fly as sportsmen and women in their own right, just as do the able-bodied, 10,000 miles and more to represent their countries at their own international sports festivals? Who would have thought that one day, this sports movement would gain the Olympic award of the Fearnley Cup for outstanding achievement in the service of the Olympic ideals, awarded by the Olympic Committee in 1956 on the occasion of the Olympic Games in Melbourne (Fig. 12)? And who would have thought that one day 1,000 paraplegic sportsmen and women representing 45 countries would join in their 21st International Stoke Mandeville Games at Heidelberg in 1972?

Sports Events

The sports events which are at present included in the Stoke Mandeville Games are archery, dartchery (a combining of darts and archery), table tennis, snooker, fencing (foil, épée and sabre),

Fig. 12   The Fearnley Cup

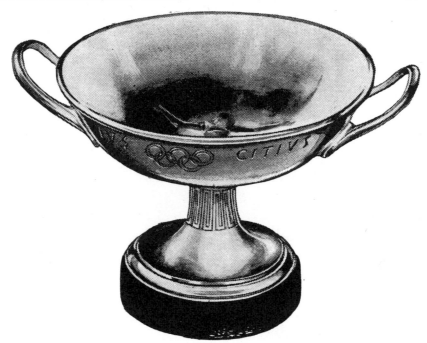

weight lifting, swimming, basketball, wheelchair dash, relay and slalom, bowling and field events (javelin throwing—distance as well as precision—shot put and discus). All these sports, with the exception of swimming and weight lifting, are carried out from the wheelchair. Other sports such as fishing, flying, and small-bore pistol shooting are also practised and, with certain groups of paraplegics, sailing, rowing and skin diving, provided adequate precautions and suitable facilities can be made available for such contests.

Standards and Aims of the Stoke Mandeville Games

As one would expect from any sports movement, the standard of performance in the various sports events has steadily improved in the course of years, and almost every year records are broken in one sport or another. Naturally, as in sport for the able-bodied, the

will to win is always strongest amongst the paralysed during national and international contests. However, any exaggerated nationalism, commercialism, or political, racial and religious discrimination is quite inconsistent with the ideals of the Games and would be abhorrent. As already pointed out, the Olympic Games have suffered greatly in recent years from commercialism, exaggerated nationalism and racialism and this has led to the bitter and cynical criticism that "international sporting contests provide an opportunity for the maximum degree of international misunderstanding in the minimum of time". Although such criticism is certainly exaggerated, there is some truth in it, and even International Sports Organisations for the Disabled are not immune from such dangers.

It cannot be emphasised too strongly that, important as the standard of athletic performance may be, the Stoke Mandeville Games have a much greater significance. They have become an annual reunion of men, women and young adults, stricken by one of the greatest tragedies of human life. Through international sport, they have come to know, understand and appreciate one another, and these Games have become the cradle of hope for thousands of others who still dwell in darkness and despair. The ideals of these Games are embodied in the symbol of three entwining wheels, which represent FRIENDSHIP, UNITY, SPORTSMANSHIP, as shown in Fig. 13. The aims of the Games are described in a message which is displayed in the Sports Hall of the Stoke Mandeville Sports Stadium for the Paralysed and other Disabled as a reminder of responsibility to all who enter:

> "The aim of the Stoke Mandeville Games is to unite paralysed men and women from all parts of the world in an international sports movement, and your spirit of true sportsmanship today will give hope and inspiration to thousands of paralysed people. No greater contribution can be made to society by the paralysed than to help, through the medium of sport, to further friendship and understanding amongst nations".

This concept is that of a movement for peace, and the ideals of the Olympics of the Paralysed are in accordance with those of Pierre de Coubertin, founder of the modern Olympics of the able-bodied.

Patronage of the Olympic Movement

Late in 1975 the author had correspondence with the International Olympic Committee, and in particular a meeting with Lord Killanin, the President of the IOC, to discuss the possibility of a closer tie between our two Organisations. As a result, the International Olympic Committee, meeting at Innsbruck during the Winter Olympics 1976, decided that the Olympic Movement will in future give its patronage to the Stoke Mandeville Paraplegic Games. This is indeed the fulfilment of a dream that our world sports movement of the paralysed would one day gain such gratifying recognition.

Classification of the Physical Handicap of the Spinal Paralysed

The higher the spinal cord injury the larger is the neurological deficit, ie. loss of motor function and sensibility, especially postural sensibility. However, the classification is made both on a functional basis and on the neurological deficit. The aim of this classification is to ensure fair play and to eliminate as far as possible injustices between participants in the same class and to give priority to the more severely disabled. For instance, a paraplegic with a low lesion, say below the 10th thoracic segment (T 10), who has developed a great deformity of the spine and has had to undergo one or several operative procedures may have to be put in a higher class on account of his or her inadequate postural control. On the other hand, paraplegics with complete lesions say at the level of T 7 or 8 who have developed great skill and good postural control, may request to compete in classes with spinal cord lesions well below their own lesion. The greatest difficulties of classification are with polio patients and incomplete traumatic paraplegics and tetraplegics suffering from partial or disseminated paralysis or weakness of muscle groups. Finally, it must also be said that some competitors may exaggerate their disability during the medical examination in order to be classified as more severely disabled than they

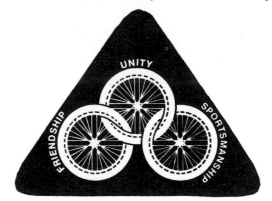

Fig. 13. The symbol of the Olympics of the Paralysed, representing Friendship, Unity and Sportsmanship.

really are. This was found particularly in wheelchair basketball and swimming. Therefore, in cases of uncertainty it is necessary for the classifying medical officer to watch the competitor's performance during the sporting events.

From all this it is clear that classification of the paralysed demands intimate knowledge and good experience on the part of the medical officer involved, whose duty it is to give guidance to his para-medical colleagues concerned with the training and education of the paralysed as well as with judging the contests.

The Executive Committee of the I S M G F has set up a panel of competent physicians and surgeons who have gained great experience in the classification of paraplegics and tetraplegics for competitive sport and Dr. Caibre McKann has compiled the findings of the panel in a memorandum.

The basis of these classifications, details of which are given in Table 2 comprises the following sub-division: 3 types of cervical lesion, 2 types of trunk lesion, 2 types of lesion limited to the lower limbs. These classifications concern all sports events with the exception of weight lifting for which the competitors are divided according to their weight. Sometimes minor modifications have been brought to the basic

TABLE 2. Classification of Para- and Tetraplegics for Competitive Sport

CERVICALS

Class 1a   Upper Cervical lesions (at and below C 6) with triceps not functional against gravity (up to and including Grade 3 of the Medical Research Council's Scale).

Class 1b   Cervical lesions below C 6/7 with good triceps, wrist extensors and flexors, but having no finger flexors or extensors of functional value (ie. below 3 M R C Scale), but good wrist extensors.

Class 1c   Lower cervical lesions (below C 8) with good triceps and strong long finger flexors and extensors to power 4 MRC Scale, but having no interossei or lumbrical musculature and abductor and opponens pollicis innervated by the first thoracic segment (T 1) of functional value. The paralysis of the interossei and lumbricals is certainly a handicap for swimmers during the adduction movements of arms and hands as the adduction of the fingers are paralysed and thus the power of propulsion may be diminished. In all cervical groups the function and strength of the muscles of the shoulder girdle (trapezius, rhomboids, latissimus dorsi and pectorals) have also to be included in the classifications. This applies in particular to sports events such as field events and swimming.

THORACIC

Class 2   Below T 1 to T 5 inclusive—having no balance when sitting.

Class 3   Below T 6 to T 10 inclusive—with ability to keep balance when sitting, ignoring non-functional lower abdominal muscles (MRC Grades 1 and 2)

Class 4   Below T 11 to L 3 inclusive—provided that quadriceps and gluteal muscle power is non-functional (MRC Grades 1 and 2)

Class 5   Below L 4 to S 2 inclusive—provided that quadriceps and gluteal function is MRC Grade 3 and above.

Class 6   Spinal injuries with minimal muscular deficit.

TESTING POINTS SYSTEM ACCORDING TO MRC SCALE
0=total lack of voluntary contraction
1=faint contraction without any result on the mobility (flicker)
2=contraction with very weak movement only, with elimination of gravity
3=contraction allowing a movement only against gravity
4=contraction allowing a movement against resistance and gravity
5=contraction allowing movement against strong resistance or movement of normal strength.

classification according to the various disciplines of the sports events.

A Points System for Lower Limb Muscle Function

In order to ensure priority of the participation of athletes with more severe physical deficit a points system was introduced for paralysed athletes for Classes 4, 5 and 6 in relation to full function of muscles of the lower limbs, as shown hereunder:

TABLE 3. Point system for severe Physical Deficit

		R.	L.
Hips:	Flexors	5	5
	Adductors	5	5
	Abductors	5	5
	Extensors	5	5
Knees:	Flexion	5	5
	Extension	5	5
Ankles:	Dorsification	5	5
	Planar flexion	5	5
		40	40 TOTAL=80

Class 4	Those between	1–20 Traumatic
		1–15 Polio
Class 5	Those between	21–40 Traumatic
		16–35 Polio
Class 6	Those between	41–60 Traumatic
		36–50 Polio

Ineligible for entry into competition
Traumatic points score 61 and above
Poliomyelitis points score 51 and above

The Rules of Sport for the Paralysed

Ever since the Stoke Mandeville Games were founded, rules for the individual sports events were introduced, following as closely as possible the international rules for the same sports in competitions for the able-bodied. Over the years, we have learned a great deal about the degree to which these rules can be adapted to the sport for the paralysed. Each year, meetings of doctors, trainers and team leaders are held immediately after the games, at which every country taking part has the opportunity of being represented and of airing its comments and suggestions in the light of the experience gained during the various events. These meetings have indeed been of great importance for adapting the rules of able-bodied sports to wheelchair sports and also for the amendment of our own rules. They formed the groundwork for a *Handbook of Rules of the Stoke Mandeville Games*, originally compiled by the author with the cooperation of his co-workers Charlie Atkinson and Joan Scruton, and later with the cooperation of Medical and Technical Sub-Committees set up by the Executive Committee and the Council of the I S M G F. These rules are now accepted world-wide by all organisations concerned with sport of the paralysed, including the International Sports Organisation for Multi-Disabled (I S O D); they are by no means rigid and can be amended or changed every four years in the light of further experience. They are now available through the generosity of Mr. Mike Markus in Johannesburg as small booklets covering most of the individual sports practised at the Stoke Mandeville Games and can be obtained from the General Secretary, I S M G F, Stoke Mandeville Sports Stadium for the Paralysed and other Disabled, Harvey Road, Aylesbury, England. It seems to be necessary, however, to summarize essential points of the rules, which has been done here in the individual sections on specific sports.

The Problem of Training Paraplegics and Tetraplegics in Sporting Activities

Clinical sport is an essential part of the general reconditioning of the spinal man despite his severe disablement to utilize and develop not only his remaining potentialities and talents but also to arouse, mobilise and develop such dormant intellectual and physical faculties as he may possess to carve out a new scheme of active and useful life. This basic philosophy of training is, of course, applicable to any other type of disablement, such as amputation, blindness and cerebral palsy with, naturally, certain modifications according to the individual disability.

The purpose of all remedial exercises in the period of re-conditioning of the paralysed is to develop a new scheme of neuro-muscular integration. These exercises should commence as soon as possible in the early stages of spinal paralysis while the patient is still confined to bed and should include sporting activities when he is able to get up and about in his wheelchair. The conclusion drawn by the famous physiologist Sir Charles Sherrington from his experimental work on animals: "Each and every part of the animal is integrative" can also be applied to man, as the author of this book has proved in his own work on the spinal man (Guttmann 1945–1973).

Physiological Aspects of the Training

The objects to be pursued are as follows:

(a) *Training of normal muscles above the level of paralysis with anatomical attachment in the paralysed area.* The old concept of neurologists and physiologists that, following transection of the spinal cord, there is no connection between the paralysed part and the normal parts of the body is certainly no longer valid.

It must be remembered that in complete spinal cord transections, even as high as the cervical cord, the paralysed part of the body still remains connected to the central nervous system above the lesion. This is accomplished through the anatomical arrangement of certain muscle groups which have their segmental innervation above the level of the cord transection, but on the other hand, are attached by their insertion points to the paralysed parts of the spine and, in particular, to the pelvis. In transection of the distal thoracic cord, the muscle groups available

for this physiological link in restoring stability of the trunk and guaranteeing the upright position are the back muscles, including the latissimus dorsi and the trapezius as well as the abdominal muscles (Guttmann 1953, 1973). In transection above the 6th dorsal segment of the cord, where motor paralysis also involves the abdominal muscles and the distal back muscles, the latissimus dorsi, with its attachment to the posterior rim of the pelvis, and the trapezius reaching down to the 12th dorsal vertebra are still available for the reconditioning of neuromuscular function in the spinal man, on account of their innervation in the cervical cord. Figure 14 shows the connection of the latissimus dorsi, innervated by the mid-cervical cord, with the paralysed part of the body in a patient with complete transection of the cord at the level of the third thoracic segment and Figure 15 demonstrates the attachment at the 12th thoracic vertebra of the trapezius muscles, innervated by the first 4 cervical segments in addition to the innervation by the accessory nerve, the 11th cranial nerve. These are the muscles on which a paraplegic with a high lesion has to rely to restore and maintain his upright position. Therefore, the purpose of exercising these muscles is to build up their strength and endurance to overcome fatigue. At the same time, it is imperative to increase the strength of the arm muscles, for, in certain sports in which normally the legs play the most essential part in the efficiency of performance (such as putting the shot, throwing the javelin or club), the paraplegic has to rely entirely on the increased power of the arm, shoulder and back muscles. How much, for instance, the able-bodied javelin thrower relies on the power of his leg and hip muscles is immediately apparent when he throws the javelin from the sitting position, as we found with British Olympic Internationals. In a contest with trained paraplegic javelin throwers who had developed a compensatory function of the arm and shoulder muscles by increasing their strength and endurance to an excessive degree, the performance of the able-bodied sportsmen

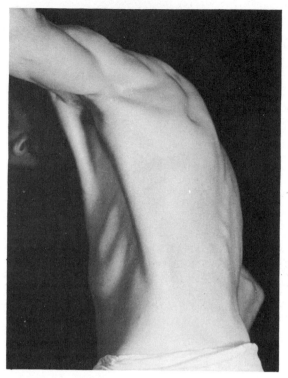

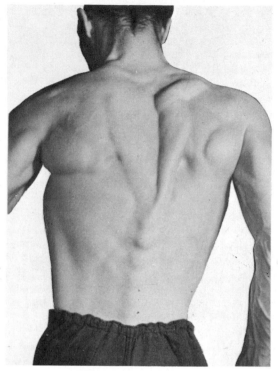

Fig. 14   Hypertrophy of the latissimus dorsi muscle in a complete paraplegic below the 3rd thoracic segment.

Fig. 15   Hypertrophy of the trunk muscles as a result of training in archery.

throwing the javelin from a sitting position was by no means superior—in fact, in most instances, it was not as good as that of the well-trained paraplegics.

From this experience, it is worth considering whether it would not improve the performance of the able-bodied athlete in field events if he were to develop his arm and shoulder muscles to a greater strength by adding training in throwing from a sitting position to the usual training in the standing position as is done at present.

So long as the patient is confined to bed, the reconditioning exercises are carried out with the aid of chest expanders, their pull-weight being gradually increased. Once the paraplegic is up in a wheelchair and attending the physiotherapy department, exercises with pulleys and weights

and swinging the paralysed body in a horizontal plane with the patient's arms extended above the head and gripping the Guthrie-Smith frame can be added.

At this stage, various sports such as weight-lifting, climbing ropes and, in particular, archery can be included in the reconditioning exercises. Progression with these exercises is gradual but continuous, and can take the form of an over-all activity in different sports each day or a number of performances of a particular sport, for instance archery, to increase the strength of the shoulder and arm muscles. The training effect of archery on shoulder and back muscles can readily be appreciated if one realizes that, in a Columbia Round, one of the first rounds practised, 24 arrows are shot at

Fig. 16 The Stoke Mandeville
Pedal Bed Cycle.

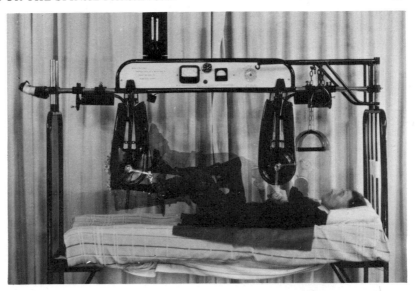

each of the distances of 50, 40 and 30 yards, with a pull-weight varying between 24 and 42 lb, according to age, sex and stage of reconditioning. In due course, the hypertrophy of the shoulder muscles increases steadily, and the degree to which this can be developed by continuous training is shown in Figure 15 which depicts the shoulder muscles of a traumatic paraplegic with a lesion below the 6th dorsal segment.

In 1946, I designed a special pedal exerciser called the Stoke Mandeville bed cycle (Fig. 16) which served two purposes in the reconditioning of paraplegics: (1) in relaxing spasticity, a common complication of spinal cord lesions above the 12th thoracic segment, by alternating passive movements of the spastic paralysed legs, and (2) by promoting self-activated exercises by the paraplegic to improve the strength of the leg muscles in incomplete lesions of the spinal cord, especially following polio or traumatic conus-cauda equina lesions, and in cervical spinal root lesions to improve the strength of biceps and triceps (Fig. 16). A full description of this apparatus has been given elsewhere (Guttmann 1973).

(b) *Development of a new pattern of postural sensibility, through By-Pass Sensory-Motor Innervation* (Guttmann 1953, 1973). A transection of the spinal cord results not only in muscular paralysis below the level of the lesion but also in loss of all forms of sensibility. As a result of the loss of postural sensibility, the higher the level of the transection of the cord the more difficult it is to maintain the equilibrium of the body in a vertical position. Therefore, a new pattern of postural sensibility has to be developed to enable the paraplegic to regain his equilibrium in a sitting position, which is one of the pre-conditions for the acquisition of athletic skill. This is achieved along the nerves of the trunk muscles mentioned above which have their segmental innervation above the cord lesion but their attachment in the paralysed part of the body—in particular, the pelvis. Afferent impulses arising from any movement of the pelvis, such as occurs when the paraplegic raises his arms when sitting, are transmitted along the nerves of these normal muscles to the spinal cord above the cord transection and from there to the cerebral centres controlling posture, which in turn set off the appropriate efferent re-

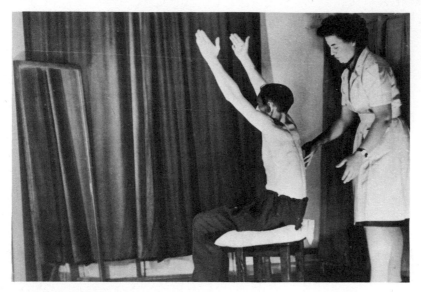

Fig. 17   Balancing exercises in front of a mirror.

sponses to the muscular system to initiate control of balance. The techniques to achieve this are, firstly, balancing exercises in front of a mirror during which the arms are raised in various directions, whereby the paraplegic learns to achieve equilibrium by visual guidance (Fig. 17).

Secondly, as soon as a new pattern of postural sensibility develops along the nerves of the normal back muscles, the paraplegic learns to sit with his arms raised and his eyes closed. Already, at this stage, archery has proved to be an excellent exercise for the restoring of posture. The third stage is keeping the equilibrium when throwing or catching a ball or heavy object, such as a sandbag. At this stage, throwing the javelin, throwing the club, and putting the shot can also be usefully employed.

The final stage in restoring the equilibrium consists of rapid alternations between free movements of the arms and body against resistance. This is practised by punchball exercises, whereby variations of movement and diversity of situations occur (Fig. 2). This is the stage of postural readjustment where table-tennis and wheelchair basketball have proved to be invaluable, for the variations of movements and diversity of situations caused by the movement of the ball on the one hand and the movement of the opponent in his wheelchair on the other are an excellent training exercise for promoting a new pattern of postural control in the paralysed (see Figs. 23–25).

Swimming has also been usefully employed for the restoration of postural control in the water in both paraplegics and tetraplegics. The paralysed part of the body, especially in higher cord lesions, has a tendency to float in the water (Figs 40 & 41), due to its greater buoyancy, and the paralysed swimmer, especially when using the breast stroke, may therefore at first experience difficulty in keeping head and shoulders above water and must learn to develop a new postural control in the water. In this connection, special mention may be made of paralysed patients in which the paralysis is combined with amputation of a limb. Such patients can be outstanding examples of the dormant mobilization of adjustment forces in the human body. The most extreme examples in this respect are patients with high lesions who were good swimmers before their injury, as the following case

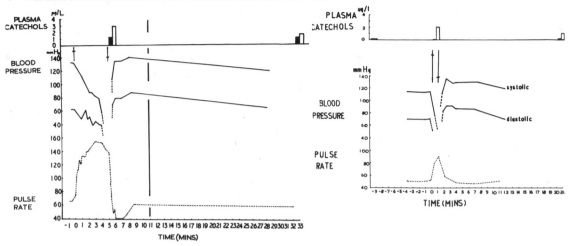

Fig. 18   Effects of tilting on blood pressure, pulse rate and catecholamines
in complete cervical lesions.

shows. A man lost his left arm in the upper third during the Second World War, and after the war developed a tranverse myelitis resulting in a complete paraplegia above the chest. He was a keen swimmer before his illness and while under treatment at Stoke Mandeville insisted on continuing this sport. At first, being a one-arm amputee and paralysed and unable to use his legs, he swam in circles like a fish with one fin. He was then fitted with a frog-arm on the stump of his left arm which enabled him to swim straight. When, after six weeks of training, the frog-arm was removed, he nevertheless was able to swim in a slightly diagonal line; indeed an excellent demonstration of the astounding sensory-motor readjustment. Another example concerns a man who sustained a fracture dislocation of his 6th cervical vertebra, resulting in a complete tetraplegia below the 7th cervical segment. At the time of his injury he was investigating the inside of a lead shot-blasting machine which was erroneously switched on, and in addition to sustaining a high spinal cord injury his left arm was severed in the upper third. During the later stages of rehabilitation, he, too, was taught to swim the back stroke, using his partially paralysed right arm and the stump of his amputated arm.

(c) *Reconditioning of the cardiovascular system* (Guttmann 1946, 1953, 1973). In the process of acquiring athletic skill in the spinal man, the reconditioning of the cardiovascular system is as important as that of muscular and sensory mechanisms. It must be remembered that, in the initial and early stages of transection of the cord, the vascular bed in the paralysed areas is deprived of its vasomotor control, as a result of the paralysis of the vaso-constrictors. This is particularly conspicuous in complete lesions above the 5th dorsal segment, where the control of the splanchnic nerve is abolished. Therefore, when the patient is raised from the horizontal to the upright position, a rapid and uninhibited accumulation of blood in the abdominal area and lower limbs occurs as a result of the inability of the blood vessels in the viscera to contract. This, in turn, results in decreased venous return and consequently insufficient cardiac output.

Since 1946, I have been engaged with my co-workers in systematic studies of the effects of postural change on the cardiovascular system in paraplegics and tetraplegics due to rapid tilting from the horizontal to the upright position (1946, 1953, 1963). As two of my co-workers, Munro and Robinson (1960), found that patients with high thoracic and cervical lesions had significantly lower levels of adrenaline and noradrenaline in the peripheral plasma than normal subjects, we also examined the effect of postural changes on plasma catecholamine levels in relation to the cardio-vascular changes in these patients. It was found that the incidence of fainting in subjects below T 5/6 was only slightly higher than in normal people submitted to the same tilting procedure. However, only a few of the spinal subjects with lesions above T 5/6, especially tetraplegics, were able to maintain consciousness for more than two or three minutes. The T 5/6 level thus appears to be critical for the maintenance of the erect posture. The reason is that considerable vasomotor regulation is still possible when the lesion is below T 6, but with lesions above this level the vasomotor centres have little control over the vascular bed. Transient compensation of the blood circulation on raising the paralysed from the horizontal to the vertical position is effected by an increase in the heart rate, but finally the lack of cardiac output results in a steep fall of blood pressure, and the vascular hypotension results in loss of consciousness. The invariable premonitory symptoms of syncope in spinal subjects are blurring and finally loss of vision, as well as giddiness and buzzing and ringing in the ears. Figure 18 a demonstrates the effect of postural change from the horizontal to the vertical position and vice versa in a tetraplegic below C 5 and a paraplegic below T 4/5, and Figure 19 shows the electrocardiographic changes. The plasma catecholamine changes of the individuals with complete spinal cord lesions who fainted showed a marked degree of inconsistency. The procedure often produced a much greater increase of adrenaline than noradrenaline in the plasma, and the total catecholamine values were usually in excess of what might be expected for the level of the lesion.

However, the initial tendency to fainting of patients with cord lesions of high level, in particular tetraplegics, gradually disappears with proper training of these patients. To overcome this maladaptation of the blood circulation to posture by redistribution of the blood-flow from the viscera and to promote the circulatory adjustments necessary to meet the metabolic requirements during athletic performances of the paraplegic and tetraplegic, exercises involving frequent change of posture combined with resistance exercises (the latter producing a squeezing effect of muscular contractions on the vascular system), as well as the application of an abdominal binder before transferring the patient from the horizontal to the upright position, have proved invaluable. The reconditioning of the ventilatory capacity of the lungs and increased respiratory power, especially a deep breath resulting in reflex vaso-constriction, may also help to improve the maladaptation of the blood circulation.

(d) *Reconditioning of the respiratory system.* In upper thoracic and cervical injuries the paralysis of the intercostal muscles, in addition to the paralysis of the abdominals, results in considerable reduction of the respiratory function. This constitutes, of course, a very serious handicap to the activities of these patients in the early stages of paralysis. The tetraplegic's ability to ventilate depends almost entirely on the diaphragm, the function of which in turn is also reduced as a result of the paralysis of the abdominal muscles.

Studies on the vital capacity of the lungs in tetraplegics (Cameron *et al.* 1955; Talbot *et al.* 1957; Wingo 1957) showed a reduction to a third of the normal and a proportionate reduction in the inspiratory and expiratory reserve volumes. This reduction is increased by raising the patient from the horizontal to the upright position. This postural effect is due to the paralysis of the abdominal muscles, especially in the early stages, which allows the intestines to bulge through the flaccid abdominal wall, the diaphragm thus assuming a lower position in the chest and resulting in smaller excursions. In tetraplegics, who, in addition to the paralysis of

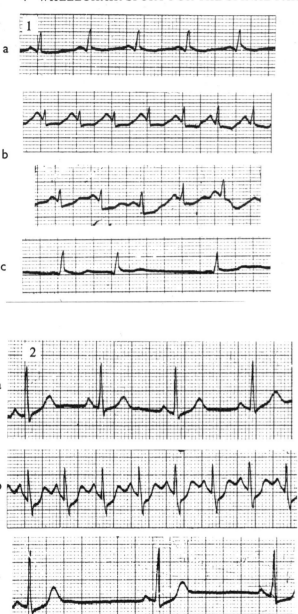

Fig. 19 Effects of tilting as shown on the electrocardiogram: *a* before tilting; *b* after tilting to a vertical position; and *c* following the return to a horizontal position. Note the reactive bradycardia.

the intercostal and abdominal muscles, have a unilateral paralysis of the diaphragm, the vital capacity may at first be as low as 0.3–0.4 litres. In due course, however, the ventilatory capacity of the tetraplegic improves, and in 1947 Gilliat, Whitteridge and I found a vital capacity of 2.8 litres and an inspiratory capacity of 2.2 litres in a tetraplegic with a complete lesion below C 6 in the later stages, tested while the man was sitting in a wheelchair. At this stage in his rehabilitation the man was able to play table-tennis, with the table-tennis bat fixed to his hand as the finger muscles were paralysed. Even in the presence of an additional unilateral paralysis of the diaphragm, the improvement of the ventilatory capacity can be considerable. One of my tetraplegic patients, aged 19, with a complete paralysis of the left diaphragm, whose vital capacity $3\frac{1}{2}$ months after injury was only 0.75 litres, improved within 195 days to 1.2 litres; 278 days after injury the vital capacity was 1.7–2 litres in a lying position and 1.3 litres sitting, which enabled him to spend most of the day in a wheelchair. He learned to control an electric typewriter with the aid of an electronic device, called POSSUM, developed in the Electro-Mechanical Laboratory of the Stoke Mandeville National Spinal Injuries Centre (Clarkson & Maling 1963), by using his mouth and blowing and sucking through a tube.

What is the mechanism underlying the improvement of the ventilatory function of the lungs in high spinal cord lesions? In the first place, in order to overcome the respiratory deficit, neck and shoulder muscles, especially the sterno-mastoid and trapezius, can be mobilized as auxiliary respiratory muscles and developed to compensate for the paralysis of the intercostal muscles to a considerable extent and thus facilitate more adequate ventilation. This reconditioning of the pulmonary function is achieved by an upwards pull of sternum and chest wall by the function of these auxiliary respiratory muscles, which increases the antero-posterior diameter of the chest. Early onset and

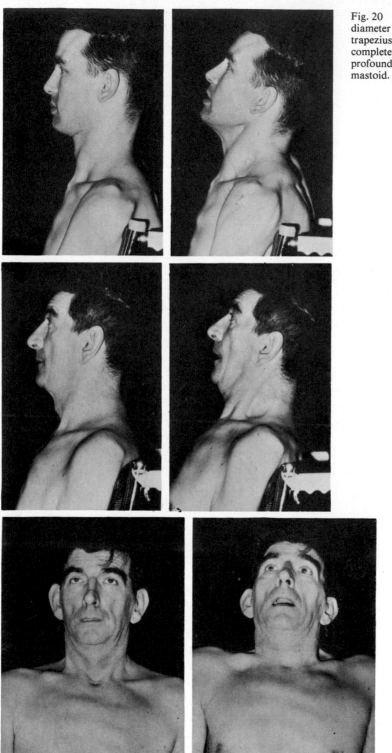

Fig. 20   Increase of antero-posterior diameter of the chest by upward pull of the trapezius and sterno-mastoid muscles in a complete Cervical 5 lesion. Note the profound hypertrophy of the sterno-mastoid.

Fig. 21   The same effect in a complete Cervical 7 lesion.

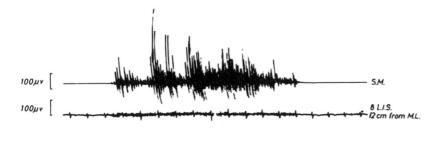

Fig. 22   Reflex activity of the 8 intercostals in comparison with the sterno-mastoid (SM) on deep inspiration 4 months after complete lesion below Cervical 3 on the left and Cervical 5 on the right. Note the much reduced action potential on the left 8th interspace due to paralysis of the diaphragm on that side.

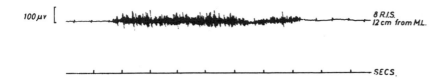

continuation of training by breathing exercises results in increased strength of these muscles. The degree of hypertrophy which can be achieved in the auxiliary respiratory muscles by systematic training can be considerable and is shown in the illustrations of two patients with complete lesions of the cervical cord. Figure 20 demonstrates the upwards pull and increase of the antero-posterior diameter of the chest achieved by the action of the shoulder muscles and, in particular, the sternomastoid during inspiration, in a case of complete transverse lesion below C 5 following fracture dislocation of the mid-cervical spine. Figure 21 shows the same effect in a case of complete lesion below C 7, following fracture dislocation of C 6 vertebra, with special reference to the function of the trapezius.

There is, however, another factor to be considered in the reconditioning of the pulmonary function in tetraplegics. In view of the fact that the paralysed intercostal and abdominal muscles regain their tone once the stage of spinal shock has subsided and the spinal cord below the level of transection, now isolated from the cerebral influences, regains its own automatic function, the question arises (Guttmann & Bell 1958) whether and to what extent the paralysed

intercostal and abdominal muscles may participate in the act of breathing by reflex action. Electro-myographic studies which I have undertaken with my former Senior Research Assistant, Dr. J. Silver, have clearly shown that, while it is difficult during the immediate stage following tetraplegia (stage of spinal shock) to record action potentials from the intercostals in response to the stimulus of breathing, the electrical response of these muscles to the act of breathing was very conspicuous once the stage of spinal shock had subsided and full reflex activity of the isolated cord had developed (Fig. 22) (Guttmann & Silver 1965). It was found that the reflex activity of the intercostals showed a rhythm pattern in close correlation to the rhythmic movements of the chest during the act of breathing. It commenced either in mid- or late inspiration and lasted until early expiration. The co-ordinated action of the paralysed intercostals is due to a stretch reflex. The diaphragm, on descending during inspiration, passively separates the lower ribs because of its anatomical attachment, thus causing a stretch effect on the intercostal muscles, which acts as an afferent stimulus to a stretch reflex. Our findings indicate that this co-ordinated reflex function also plays a part in the process of respiratory re-conditioning. The intercostal muscles, having re-gained their tone once the spinal shock has sub-sided, restore by their reflex contractions the tension and rigidity of the intercostal spaces which are essential for a more powerful function of the diaphragm and thus contribute to a better ventilation of the lungs. It can be assumed that the improved ventilatory capacity of the lungs resulting from the compensatory function of the auxiliary respiratory muscles on the one hand and the rhythmic reflex contractions of the inter-costal muscles on the other, increases the circu-latory filling pressure of the pulmonary vascular system, which in turn contributes to the recondi-tioning of the cardio-vascular system by increas-ing the venous return to the heart with conse-quent increased cardiac output. This is another reason why the initial tendency to fainting when the patient is raised from the horizontal to the vertical position disappears in the course of training, thus enabling these patients to start an active life and take part in sports competitions, such as archery, table tennis and swimming.

Acquisition by the Paralysed of Athletic Skill
in Specific Sports

The acquisition of athletic skill in specific sports by the spinal man is a complex process of adaptation and re-adjustment in order to achieve the highest possible degree of neuro-muscular integration which enables him to reach top-level performances. Various factors have to be taken into consideration which include the following:

1. *Type and Severity of the Remaining Disability*

In spinal cord afflictions, whether traumatic or non-traumatic, one has to distinguish between complete and incomplete lesions and the level of the lesion, i e. whether it affects only the lower limbs or also includes the abdominal and trunk muscles or parts of the upper limbs, and furthermore whether the paralysis is of a spastic or a flaccid nature. Other factors to be considered are the degree of loss of postural sensibility and its effect on the patient's equilibrium in a vertical position and the disturbance of vasomotor control in injuries above the 5th thoracic segment. Patients with complete or severe incomplete lesions are chairbound, while in less severe incomplete lesions standing and walking capabilities may be preserved or restored. Accordingly, the training will differ considerably.

2. *Intelligent Adaptation of Types of Sport to the Disability*

This is of particular importance to tetraplegics and also to combined disabilities such as are described in the case of arm amputation and high paraplegia. (See also the chapter on weightlifting.)

3. *Adaptation of the Rules of Sports of the Able-bodied to the Needs of the Paralysed.*

This has already been discussed in the section on classification in Chapter 4.

Clinical sport as a supplement to conventional methods of remedial exercises has proved invaluable in the process of over-all reconditioning in achieving the highest possible degree of neuro-muscular integration in the spinal man.

It was only to be expected that, in due course and according to aptitude and inclination, paraplegics would acquire athletic skill in specific sports. Already during the period of preparatory training the physical instructor will discover the patient's aptitude for a specific sport and will encourage him to take it up as recreation after discharge from hospital. It will be seen, therefore, that there is no strict or dogmatic division between the period of reconditioning and the commencement of training for the acquisition of athletic skill in a specific sport.

The principles of acquiring athletic skill in specific sports for paraplegics do not differ from those for able-bodied sportsmen. They consist of the training of specific movement-patterns to achieve the highest possible degree of efficiency of performance, the only difference being that in paraplegics these movement-patterns are confined to the head, trunk and upper limbs and they differ also in terms of strength and endurance as well as of range and direction, as there are greater limitations of potential with the paralysed in comparison with the able-bodied. For instance, the movement-patterns in training for distance javelin throwing differ considerably from those for precision javelin throwing. While the former demands powerful movements of the

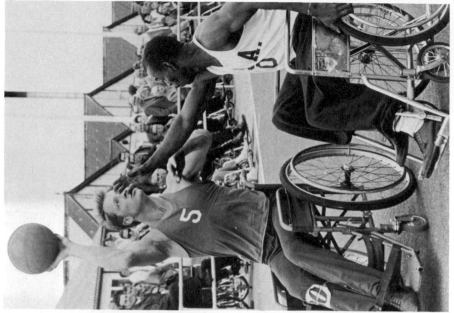

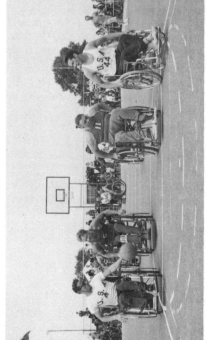

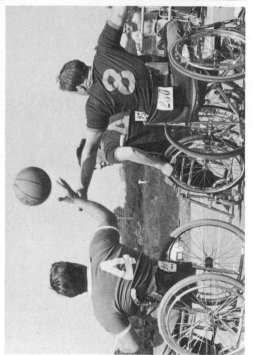

Fig. 24   Attempting to intercept a pass.

Fig. 23   Scenes during a basketball match, demonstrating the various actions and postures of the players.

whole trunk, shoulder and arm, the latter requires a more discriminating movement of the shoulder joint and wrist, similar to the movement pattern in dart-throwing. Still different are the techniques of movement patterns for shot putting and club and discus throwing from the chair. Common to all the five field events mentioned is the necessity to train the paraplegic to maintain his equilibrium in his wheelchair before, during and after completing the throw without affecting its power and direction. In swimming, which has become very popular with paraplegics, training, in addition to improving endurance, is directed to the development of movement patterns which promote, as already mentioned, a new postural control in the water.

The most dramatic effects of training in the acquisition of specific athletic skill can be seen in basketball. In this sport, the spinal man can attain degrees of neuro-muscular integration and postural control which must be seen to be believed. It is true to say that the man and his wheelchair have become one, like the rider and his mount in polo. He has learned the techniques of passing, catching, dribbling, shooting and intercepting the ball while racing along the court in his wheelchair, at the same time trying to avoid crashing into an opponent's chair, which would be regarded immediately as a foul. It is sometimes quite breathtaking for the spectator to see a paraplegic racing along at high speed, catching the ball with one hand from a long pass and at the same time controlling his moving chair with the other hand, without losing direction; or to see a player at full speed scooping up the running ball from the ground with one hand and at the same time turning his chair in the direction of goal. These are only two examples which demonstrate the effect of training exercises in acquiring specific athletic skill for individual sports in paraplegics (Figs. 23–25).

The most important sports practised by spinal paraplegics and tetraplegics are now described

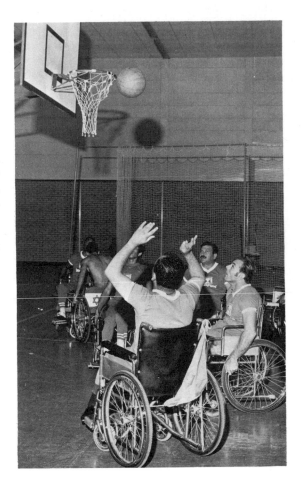

Fig. 25   The Israeli team attempts to shoot a basket.

in detail, including equipment and the essentials of the rules.

SPECIFIC SPORTS

ARCHERY

Archery has a history almost as old as man, but although man created archery out of the need to survive, today it represents one of the finest and healthiest pastimes. Our use of the bow and arrow as a means of competitive sport and re-laxation is a far cry from the day of the lion-hunting King Assur-Bani-Pal of Assyria and the days of Hastings, Crécy and Agincourt, where the bow was used as a deadly weapon in battle. Possibly the earliest representation of an archer in England is the Norman rock drawing of an archer scratched into the wall of Colchester Castle in Essex. Archery was for many cen-turies the most popular sport in England. According to Elizabeth Sheppard Jones, a former patient of Stoke Mandeville, who wrote an interesting article *Archery Historically Speaking* (1949) in *The Cord*, King Edward III went so far as to command the general practice of archery on Sundays and holidays, while other sports were forbidden, and King Henry VIII passed an act ordering any person who had reached the age of 24 to shoot at no mark less than 220 yards distant!

Archery was introduced at Stoke Mandeville as one of the first competitive sports for men, women and children and has become very popu-lar amongst paraplegics and other physically handicapped people of both sexes all over the world. Indeed, it is an ideal sport for the dis-abled from various points of view:

1. As pointed out in the section in Chapter 4 covering the physiological aspects of training, it has a profound therapeutic value for the development of the muscles of the arms and those muscles of the trunk and shoulder which guarantee the upright position of the patient, and in particular

has proved invaluable for paraplegics with middle and higher thoracic lesions, as well as cervical, lesions.

2. It has a beneficial effect on respiratory and cardio-vascular functions in para-plegics with high lesions.

3. It offers great variety in application, as the amount of exercise taken can be varied by increasing the pull weight of the bow and by shooting greater distances.

4. It has great fascination, as the archer accomplishes everything by his own judge-ment and strength and very little is mechanised for him.

5. Last, but by no means least, archery is the ideal sport in which the paraplegic and the amputee can compete with the able-bodied on equal terms. Competitions be-tween archery clubs and patients of Stoke Mandeville Spinal Centre have become a customary event.

Who could have thought in 1948, when, after training, paraplegics were just able to compete in a Columbia Round, that the time would come when a competition in the internationally accepted F I T A Round would be as possible for paraplegic archers as for the able-bodied? Who could have thought that the time would come when paraplegics would join archery clubs of the able-bodied and become master bowmen in these clubs and that a paraplegic archer would be entered in an international competition of champions to represent her country, as was the case with Mrs. Margaret Harriman of South Africa, who took up archery for the first time when a patient of Stoke Mandeville? (Fig. 26). She came 8th out of 48 competitors at an inter-national championship contest in Oslo.

Even tetraplegics with paralysis of all fingers but with good function of the extensors of the wrist can take part in and enjoy this sport. Those who have functioning triceps are pro-vided with a glove to hold the hand onto the bow; those without functioning triceps are sup-plied, in addition, with an extension splint on

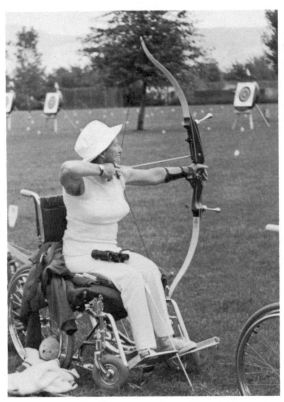

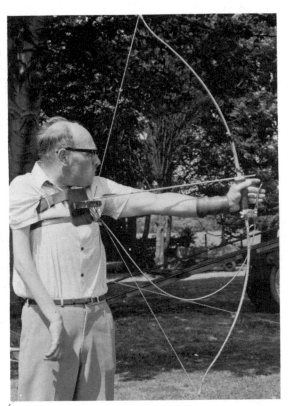

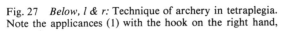

Fig. 26 *Upper left*: Mrs. Margaret Harriman, a World Champion, in an archery contest.

Fig. 27 *Below, l & r:* Technique of archery in tetraplegia. Note the applicances (1) with the hook on the right hand,

Fig. 28 *Upper, right*: Specially-adapted aids for a one-armed archer (his right arm is completely paralysed).

as all fingers are paralysed, and (2) to fix the paralysed fingers of the left hand onto the bow.

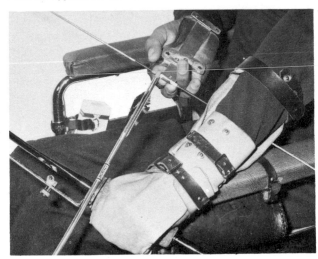

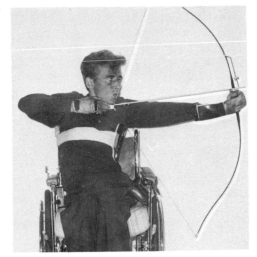

the forearm. The drawing hand is provided with a slightly curved hook of light metal on the palmar surface of the glove fitted to the palm of the hand. With the aid of these appliances, the bow string can be drawn back and then, by twisting the hand, the hook is released from the bow string, thus releasing the arrow (Fig. 27). Although tetraplegics start, like paraplegic beginners, with the easiest round, called the Tetraplegic Round (36 arrows each at 50 and 30 metres), by intensive training they succeed in shooting longer distances and some of them even the F I T A Round. Tetraplegics with complete lesions have to be strapped to the chair to maintain their equilibrium during shooting. Even disabled people with complete paralysis (or amputation) of one arm can enjoy archery by using special gadgets fixed around their chests and attached to the bow as shown in Figure 28.

The question arises of which muscles of the arms and trunk are mainly involved in archery. This problem has been studied electro-myographically on paralysed subjects with complete spinal cord lesions at levels ranging from C 6 to T 12, to ascertain the alternating muscle groups involved during the various actions in the archery exercise (Guttmann & Mehra, 1973). Surface electrodes were applied to the following muscles using a four-channel electromyograph furnished with photographic equipment: Trapezius (TRAP), Rhomboids (RHOM), Latissimus dorsi (LATDO), Pectoralis major (PECT), Serratus anterior (SERR), Deltoid (DLT), Biceps (BIC) and Triceps (TRIC).

In the course of archery exercises four actions were studied:
1. Nocking the arrow onto the bow.
2. First Draw (ID), pulling the bow string one or two inches to establish the right position for shooting (Fig. 29 upper left).
4. Horizontal Draw (FDH). The holding arm (the left) is raised to the horizontal and the bow string is pulled with the opposing arm to full extension (Fig. 29 lower left).
3. Vertical Draw (FDV). The arm holding the

bow is raised over the horizontal and the bow string is drawn to full extent with the opposing arm (Fig. 29 upper right). The arm is then lowered towards the target.
5. Releasing the Arrow (Fig. 29 lower right).

Two of the tetraplegic subjects studied had an extension splint applied to the left elbow because of paralysis of the triceps.

Figure 30 (p. 54) demonstrates the electrical activity of the individual muscles in the thoracic lesions as compared with the cervical lesions involved in the archery exercises. There was, as one would expect, great variation in the intensity of action potentials and every one of the subjects exhibited different degrees of electrical discharge whatever the level of the lesion. However, there was some uniformity in other respects: (a) the lowest electrical discharge occurred during loading and first draw, while the maximal electrical discharge was found during the full horizontal and vertical draws; (b) a sudden sharp and maximal increase of wave form as a rebound phenomenon occurred in all muscles concerned on release of the bowstring, before the electrical discharge slowed and ceased (Fig. 31 p. 55); (c) another uniformity was found in the low level or even absence of electrical discharge of the latissimus dorsi, serratus anterior and pectoralis major with the exception of one subject with a C 7 lesion where the right pectoralis major exhibited a high level of electrical activity.

In evaluating the results further, it appeared that certain muscles showed a preponderance of activity during archery and this applies in particular to the deltoid on both sides when securing the arms in a horizontal and a vertical position. That the biceps on the drawing right arm (in the right-handed subjects) and the left triceps on holding the bow in extension show high electrical discharge is obvious. However, in two cervicals supplied with extension splints because of paralysis of the triceps, the electrical discharge

Fig. 29 *Facing, left to right:* The various phases of archery technique.

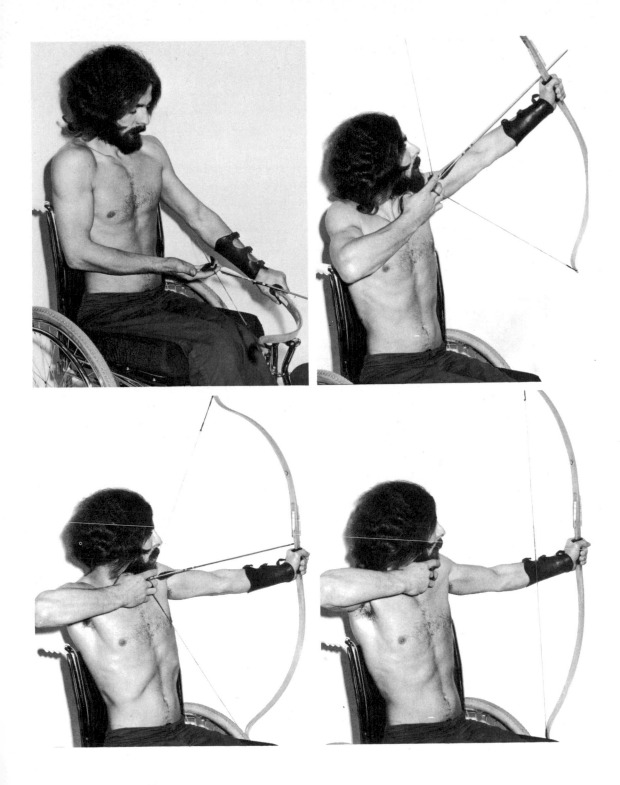

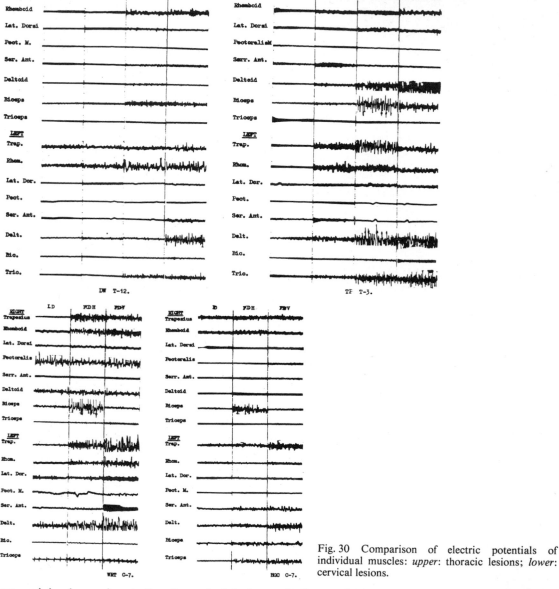

Fig. 30 Comparison of electric potentials of individual muscles: *upper*: thoracic lesions; *lower*: cervical lesions.

was minimal, or absent. In all cervical lesions and also in the T 3 lesion, trapezius and rhomboids showed particularly marked electrical activity as compared with the T 12 lesion. This indicates the importance of these muscle groups in bracing the shoulders in these high lesions (Fig. 32 p. 56).

In conclusion, this study has been useful in

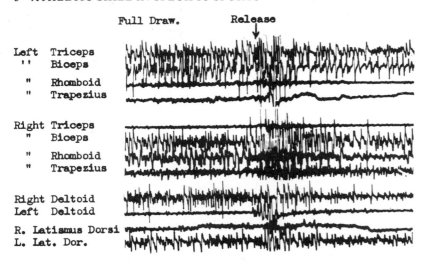

Fig. 31   Electrical rebound phenomenon on the release of the bowstring before slowing down of electrical discharge.

clarifying the activity of the muscle groups mainly involved in the various phases of archery. It was of particular interest to find that of the trunk muscles, latissimus dorsi and serratus anterior, in contrast to trapezius and rhomboids, play little part, if any, in this type of sport.

Training

The right-handed individual holds the bow in his left hand and draws the string with his right; for the left-handed, the technique, naturally, is reversed. The pre-conditions for becoming an expert archer are (a) complete mastery of the five basic components of archery technique: position, nocking, drawing, holding, and loosing; and (b) continuous practice.

The following methods refer to the use of steel or glass-fibre bows, as in the various types of laminated bows the technique has to be developed individually.

1. *Position.* The body and chair should be squarely at right angles to the shooting line or target. The bow should be held in the left hand with the knuckle at the base of the thumb towards the string. This position can be checked by holding the bow out at arm's length and placing the thumb along the outside edge of the upper limb of the bow whilst holding the bow in the fingers by the handle. The thumb is then placed round the handle without altering the position of the fingers. This ensures that when the bow is drawn the weight of the bow is taken against the pad at the base of the thumb, thus preventing the wrist from turning inwards and consequent bruising of the forearm, as well as preventing deflection of the string. When the bow is in this position, it should just rest on the knee. A brace is worn on the bow forearm as a precaution against bruising.

2. *Nocking.* This is the technique of placing the arrow in the bow so that the shaft rests on the arrow ledge and the nock of the arrow on the nocking point of the string. This is done by taking the arrow in the right hand, pile end away from the body, sliding the arrow into the bow from underneath the bow and up between the string and the bow, so that the shaft rests on the ledge, and then drawing the nock back onto the nocking point on the string. When an arrow with three fletches is used, the cock feather (i e. the feather set at right angles to the nock and usually of a different colour) should always be on the outside.

3. *Drawing.* Three fingers are used in the draw, the first finger being placed above the

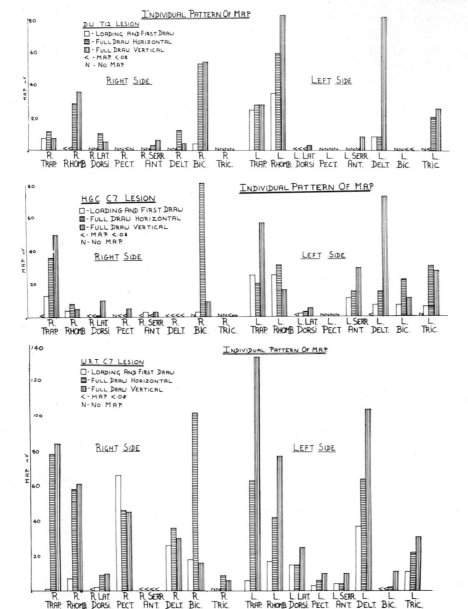

Fig. 32 Muscle groups involved in archery exercises.

arrow but not touching it and the next two fingers together below the arrow. The arrow should never be gripped between the fingers as this causes it to be deflected on release. The fingers should not be tightly curled round the string but level on the string so that the pull is taken evenly on each finger. The drawing hand and arm should be in one continuous line, i e.

the wrist must not be flexed. The draw should be made in one smooth movement, with the left hand pushing and the right hand pulling, so that both hands come up to the full-draw position together. In this full-draw position, the bow hand should be straight out towards the target and the drawing arm with the fingers evenly pulling on the string in a position underneath the side of the jaw, string touching the centre of the chin and the right arm being a continuation of the line of the arrow and the right elbow in line with the shoulder.

A finger tab or glove is used on the drawing fingers to prevent soreness.

4. *Holding.* When the full draw has been reached, a brief pause should be made to check all the points of technique of hold, draw, arm, etc., and to perfect the aim. This does not mean that the hold should be relaxed in any way, or the arrow will creep forward and result in a low hit on the target. The weight of the bow should be transferred to the shoulders, the drawing forearm being pulled back against the biceps.

5. *Loosing.* This is an art which must be perfected in order not to upset the aim or deflect the arrow. The string must slide gradually off the fingers, the fingers on no account being snatched or jerked off the string. Loosing should be a relaxed, almost unconscious movement of the drawing fingers, permitting the string to go forward and propel the arrow forward without any deflection. Having released the arrow, both hands should remain perfectly still until the arrow has hit the target, for if the hands start to fall away before the arrow hits the target, there will be a tendency for them to do so before the arrow is clear of the bow, with a resulting deflection of the arrow (Fig. 29; Fig 33).

For the first few attendances, the pupil should get used to the feel of the bow, practising drawing and holding without an arrow but *not attempting to release.* In every practice session each fault must be corrected as it arises. Failure to do this can result in low scores at a later stage which, if the pupil has been practising archery for any length of time, can be very discouraging and perhaps result in his giving up the sport. Faults which remain uncorrected at an early stage are very difficult to correct later on.

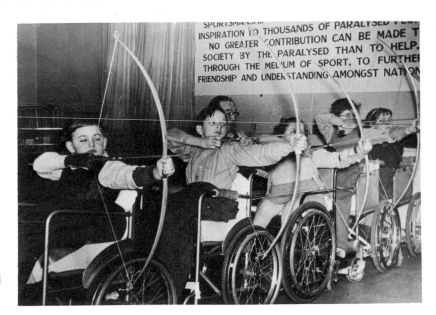

Fig. 33 Training children in archery at the National Spinal Injuries Centre, Stoke Mandeville Hospital.

As soon as the pupil has mastered the hold, draw, holding, and release, the use of the sight is taught. This will be discussed later in the rules.

The pupil is taught as soon as possible how to string and unstring a bow. The technique for a paraplegic differs from that for the able-bodied and is on the following lines: one end of the bow is fixed in the wheel or foot rest with the bow held away from the chair. One hand grasps the handle, pushing the bow away, while the other hand holding the string slides up the upper limb and slips the loop over the end of the bow. This procedure is reversed for unstringing.

During the period of training, blind shooting should also play an important part. For this, the pupil is taken to a short range, where he goes through the normal technique as for the full draw and with eyes closed practises the hold and release. This is done so that the pupil develops the feel of these actions and can tell immediately if he is doing anything wrong.

Attention to scoring should not be predominant during training, the important thing being to concentrate on technique. It is not of primary importance at this stage that the arrows should hit the gold, but they should form a compact grqup on the target. For it is comparatively easy, once having all the arrows grouped together, to move that group to the desired gold by altering the sighting.

When commencing archery, great care should be taken not to use a bow that has too heavy a poundage, as this will soon tire the pupil with the discouraging result that after a few ends the arrows will begin to drop or be scattered on the target. A qualified coach or instructor should pay particular attention to this point, as it is neither clever nor a sign of strength to use a larger bow when a bow of lower poundage will reach the desired distances just as well.

The pupil should always bear the following in mind. Complete mastery of technique is important and can be achieved only by constant practice and immediate correction of faults. No arrow should be drawn in a bow or released except from the shooting line and then only when

the signal to do so has been given. Courtesy should be shown to others on the shooting line by not talking or distracting their attention whilst shooting and by not attempting to move off the line whilst shooting is in progress. No bow should be drawn or the string released without an arrow in the bow.

TABLE 4. Distances for Competitions.

Rounds

1. Novices and Tetraplegic Rounds

36 arrows at 50 m

36 arrows at 30 m
122 cm target; 1–10 scoring

(A novice is defined as an archer who has practised archery from a wheelchair for one year or less.)

2. Short Metric Round

36 arrows at 50 m

36 arrows at 30 m
80 cm target; 1–10 scoring

3. Advanced Metric Round

Men

36 arrows at 70 m — 122 cm target 1–10 scoring

36 arrows at 50 m

36 arrows at 30 m
80 cm target 1–10 scoring

Women

36 arrows at 60 m — 122 cm target 1–10 scoring

36 arrows at 50 m

36 arrows at 30 m
80 cm target 1–10 scoring

4. Four-Day International F I T A Round

First Day. Commence shooting first part of P I T A Round.

	Women	Men
6 sighter arrows at	70 m	90 m
36 arrows at	70 m	90 m
36 arrows at	60 m	70 m
	Target: 122 cm	
	10 zone	

Second Day. Completion of the first F I T A Round.

	Women	Men
6 sighter arrows at	50 m	50 m
36 arrows at	50 m	50 m

36 arrows at   30 m   30 m
                         Target: 80 cm
                                  10 zone

Third Day. First part of second F I T A Round
                      Women Men
6 sighter arrows at   70 m   90 m
36 arrows at   70 m   90 m
36 arrows at   60 m   70 m
                       Target: 122 cm
                              10 zone

Fourth Day. Completion of the second F I T A Round
                      Women Men
6 sighter arrows at   50 m   50 m
36 arrows at   50 m   50 m
36 arrows at   30 m   30 m
                       Target: 80 cm
                              10 zone

In each of the above rounds there are individual competitions for men and women and a team competition in which the best three scores (men or women) count. FITA Rules of shooting apply. *FITA Round.* This is the International FITA, 4-Day round and is held on the first four days of the Games. Practice targets are made available at all distances on the tournament ground.

General Rules

All archers must shoot from a wheelchair.

No competitor may enter more than one round. Competitors must at all times during archery keep their feet on the foot rest. No team is allowed to enter more than three women and three men in any one round.

FITA Rules

The shooting is in one direction only and commences with the longest distance and finishes at the shortest distance in the order laid down for the competition.

Target Faces

Two standard circular FITA Target faces are used, 122 cm and 80 cm in diameter. Both these faces are divided into five concentric colour zones arranged from the Centre outwards as follows: Gold (Yellow), Red, Light Blue, Black and White.

Each colour is in turn divided by a thin line into two zones of equal width, thus making in all ten scoring zones of equal width measured from the Centre of the Gold, 6.1 cm on the 122-cm target face and 4 cm on the 80-cm target face.

Such dividing lines, and any dividing lines which may be used between colours, shall be made entirely within the higher scoring zone in each case.

Any line marking the outermost edge of the White shall be made entirely within the scoring zone.

The width of the thin dividing lines as well as the outermost line shall not exceed 2 mm on both the 122-cm and 80-cm target faces.

The centre of the target face is termed the Pinhole and shall be indicated by a small X (cross) the lines of which shall not exceed 2mm.

Target faces shall be made of paper, cloth or any other suitable material. All faces shall be uniform and of the same material.

Size of Target Face at Different Distances

For distances of 90, 70 and 60 m, the target face of 122 cm is used.

For distances of 50 and 30 m, the target face of 80 cm is used. The size of the buttress, whether round or square, must be in excess of 122 cm in any direction to ensure that any arrow hitting the buttress and cutting the outermost edge of the target face remains in the buttress.

TABLE 5. Scoring Values.

FITA Round		Colours	
Zone	Inner 10	Gold/Yellow	
	Outer 9		
	Inner 8	Red	All colours
	Outer 7		must conform to
	Inner 6	Light Blue	the set notation
	Outer 5		on the Munsell
	Inner 4	Black	colour scale.
	Outer 3		
	Inner 2	White	
	Outer 1		

Range Layout

The Range is squared off and each distance accurately measured from a point vertically beneath the Gold of each target to the shooting line. A waiting line is indicated at least 5 m behind the shooting line. Each buttress is set up at an angle of about 15°.

The centre of the Gold shall be 130 cm above the ground. A tolerance of measurement shall not exceed 5 cm.

The women's portion of the field shall be separated from the men's portion of the field by at least 5 m.

Each buttress shall be numbered. The numbers shall be 30 cm square and shall be black figures on a yellow background, alternating with yellow figures on a black background.

Points on the shooting line directly opposite each buttress shall be marked and numbered correspondingly.

Lines at right angles to the shooting line and extending from the shooting line to the target line, making lanes to contain one, two or three buttresses, may be laid down.

Shooting Equipment

A bow of any type may be used provided it subscribes to the accepted principle and meaning of the word bow as used in Target Archery in the FITA Rules.

The bow string may have a centre serving to accommodate the drawing fingers, a nocking point to which may be added servings to fit the arrow nock as necessary, and to locate this point one or two nock locators may be positioned. In addition one attachment which may not exceed a diameter of 1 cm in any direction, is permitted on the string to serve as a lip or nose mark. The serving on the string must not reach above the point of the archer's nose.

A bow string must not in any way offer aid in aiming through peephole marking or any other means.

An arrow rest which can be adjustable, an arrowplate, and a draw check indicator may all be used on the bow provided they are not electric or electronic and do not offer any additional aid in aiming.

A bowsight attached to the bow may allow for windage adjustment as well as elevation setting for aiming. It shall not incorporate a prism or lens or other magnifying device, levelling or electric device, nor shall it provide for more than one sighting point.

A bowmark in pencil-tape or any other marking material may be made on the bow for aiming. A plate or tape with distances marked may be mounted on the bow but must not offer any additional aid.

A point of aim on the ground in the shooting lane between the shooting line and target may not exceed a diameter of 7.5 cm and not protrude above the ground more than 15 cm.

Stabilisers on the bow are permitted if they do not serve as a string guide, touch anything but the bow, or present an obstacle to other archers' places on the shooting line. They shall not exceed four.

Arrows of any type may be used as long as they conform to the meaning of arrow in Target Archery. Each archer's arrows shall be marked with the archer's name or insignia and shall have the same colour(s) in fletching.

Finger protection in the form of finger stalls or tips, gloves, shooting tab or tape to draw, hold back and release the string are permitted provided they are smooth with no device to help and/or release the string. A separator between the fingers to prevent pinching may be used. On the bow hand an ordinary glove, mitten or similar may be worn.

Field glasses, telescopes and other visual aids may be used between shots for spotting arrows.

Spectacles. Shooting spectacles with lenses normally used and sun glasses are allowed but must not be marked in any way or fitted with microhole lenses.

Miscellaneous Equipment

Visual signals (green, amber and red), or plates 120 cm × 80 cm marked on one side in alternating black and yellow stripes 20–25 cm wide at an angle of 45° to the ground, with the reverse side yellow. These are used to control the shooting.

A device to indicate the order of shooting to competitors.

A large scoreboard for progressive totals after each end.

A large scoreboard for displaying the progressive scores of competitors after each distance.

Flags of light material and yellow in colour to serve as wind indicators above the centre of each target.

Range Control and Safety

A Field Captain is appointed to control the shooting and observance of the 2½-minute time limit for shooting an end of three arrows and to be responsible for safety precautions.

One blast of the whistle will be the signal for shooting to start.

Two blasts of the whistle signal the designated scorers and retrievers to go forward.

A series of blasts is the signal for all shooting to cease.

One blast is the signal for shooting to commence again.

Two Field Officers shall be appointed to work with the Field Captain.

Under the Field Captain's control two ends only of three sighter arrows are permitted preceding the commencement of shooting each day.

No archer may draw his bow, with or without an arrow, except when standing on the shooting line.

If an archer, whilst drawing his bow with an arrow before shooting starts or during break between distances, looses an arrow, intentionally or otherwise, such an arrow shall count as part of his quota of arrows for the distance to be shot, but shall not be scored even if it hits the target.

An archer who arrives after shooting has started shall forfeit the number of arrows already shot, unless the Field

Captain is satisfied that he was delayed by circumstances beyond his control.

The Field Captain has authority to extend the 2½-minute time limit in exceptional circumstances.

Shooting

Each archer shoots his arrows in ends of three arrows each.

The maximum time allowed for an archer to shoot an end of three arrows shall be 2½ min. Any arrow not shot in this period will be forfeited. Any arrow shot in excess will forfeit the highest scoring arrows of that end. If a string breaks or equipment adjustment is necessary extra time may be given.

An arrow is not deemed to have been shot if the archer can touch it with his bow.

Whilst an archer is on the shooting line he shall receive no assistance or information by word or otherwise, from anyone, other than for the purpose of making essential changes in equipment.

Scoring

One scorer shall be appointed to each target.

At 90, 70, and 60 min World Championships, scoring shall take place after every second end. In other tournaments scoring may take place after each end of three arrows or after every second end.

At 50 and 30 m, scoring shall always take place after each end of 3 arrows.

Scorers enter the value of each arrow on score sheets. Only arrows scoring ten points shall be referred to as Golds.

Neither the arrows nor the face shall be touched until all the arrows on the target have been recorded.

An arrow shall be scored according to the position of the shaft in the target face.

If more than three arrows (or six as the case may be) belonging to the same archer, should be found on the target or ground in the shooting lanes, only the three or six lowest in value shall be scored.

Should an archer repeat this he may be disqualified.

If the shaft of an arrow touches two colours or any dividing line between scoring zones, that arrow shall score the higher value of the zones affected.

Unless all arrow holes are suitably marked on each occasion when arrows are scored and drawn from the target, arrows rebounding from the target face shall not be scored.

When a rebound occurs the archer concerned, after shooting his three arrows, shall hold his bow above his head as a signal to the Field Captain and Technical Commission who will judge the hit.

An arrow hitting another arrow in the nock and remaining embedded therein, shall score according to the value of the arrow struck.

An arrow hitting another arrow and then hitting the target face shall score as it lies in the target.

An arrow hitting another arrow, and then rebounding from the target shall score the value of the struck arrow, provided the damaged arrow can be indentified.

An arrow hitting the target face after rebounding off the ground shall not score.

An arrow hitting a target other than an archer's own target, shall not score.

Score Sheets shall be signed by the Scorer and the archer, denoting that the archer agrees with the score and thereafter he may make no claim for any alteration of the score.

In the event of a tie in score the results shall be determined as follows:

For Individuals. The archer, of those tying, with the greatest number of scoring hits. If this is also a tie, then the archer of those so tying with the greatest number of Golds (hits scoring 10 points).

If this is also a tie, then the archer of those so tying with the greatest number of his scoring 9 points.

If this is also a tie, then the archers so tying shall be declared equal.

For Teams. The team, of those tying, having the archer making the highest individual score.

If this is also a tie, then the team of those so tying having the archer making the second highest individual score.

If this is also a tie, then the teams so tying shall be declared equal.

Technical Commission

There shall be appointed a Technical Commission consisting of at least five members. The Organising Committee shall appoint the Chairman of the TC who shall be an International Judge. The other four members shall be appointed by the Team Captains in a meeting preceding the tournament.

No two members of the TC shall belong to the same member organisation.

The Duties of the TC are to: Check all distances, dimensions, height of centres of targets and angles of buttresses.

Check all competitors' equipment.

Check conduct of the shooting.

Check conduct of the scoring.

Handle any disputes.

With the Field Captain, interrupt shooting because of weather, accident etc., but ensure if possible that each day's programme is completed on that day.

Consider complaints from Team Managers.

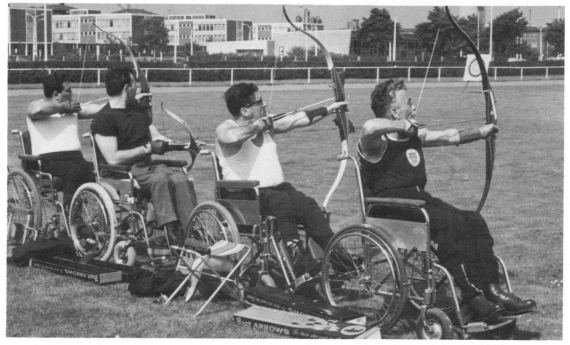

Fig. 34   *Above*: Archery competition during Stoke Mandeville Games.

Fig. 35   *Below, left*: Dartchery target.

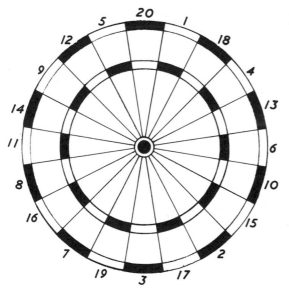

Fig. 36   *Below right*: Dartchery competition at the Stoke Mandeville Games.

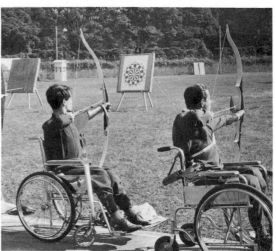

Records

TABLE 6. Records achieved in Archery.

ROUND	1970		RECORD	
	MEN	WOMEN	MEN	WOMEN
Double FITA	2113	2239	2303	2239
Advanced Metric*			833	815
Short Metric*			548	504
Tetraplegic Metric*			566	485

introduced in 1974

	MEN	WOMEN
World Record (Able-Bodied) Double FITA	2528	2424
British Record (Able-Bodied) Double FITA	2386	2313

The records achieved in 1968 by Mrs Harriman (South Africa) and in 1974 by Schmidberger (Germany) still stand.

DARTCHERY

This is a sport originally designed for paraplegics. It represents a combination of archery and darts. While the pattern of the target is that of a dart board, the shooting is done with bow and arrows instead of darts (Figs. 34–36). Therefore, the distance from the face of the target is greater than in the game of darts. Dartchery has gained increasing interest amongst paraplegics —the more so as it can be carried out in a much smaller area than can archery. As a rule, paraplegics take up dartchery once they have gained proficiency in archery, and the only difference in training is in the aiming.

Competition Rules

Competitors compete in pairs, there being competitions for men's, women's and mixed pairs. A Dartchery Face size 91.44 cm is used, scoring area size 76.2 cm (Fig. 35). The Target is fixed in such a way that the centre of the bull is 130 cm from the ground. The shooting distance is 15 m from the face of the target measured horizontally. The shooting line has to be marked. The Captains toss for start and the players shoot alternately. A shoot consists of 3 arrows, except where a game is finished in less. Arrows can-

not be re-shot and arrows which cut a line or lines of the target score value to be determined by the judge. The game is to score exactly 501, and each pair's score must start and finish with a double (the narrow outer ring). Scoring is by the subtraction method, so that the number required for the game is always shown. The inner bull (50) counts as a double of the outer bull (25). If the number required for the game is exceeded in the course of a shoot the shoot ceases and no account is taken of the score obtained during that shoot.

The rules regarding mechanical releases and devices to be used on wheelchairs are the same as in archery.

SWIMMING

The employment of water for the well-being of the individual is as old as man himself. The beneficial and recreational value of being immersed in the medium of water is already apparent in the joyful kicking of a baby, and it is later displayed by young and old in competitive and non-competitive activities in swimming pools, rivers and the sea (Guttmann 1967, 1973; Bleasdale 1975).

The introduction of swimming, in the form of hydrotherapy, as part of the clinical treatment in spinal centres and general rehabilitation centres has proved most beneficial in helping the severely disabled to master their physical deficit and give hope and confidence for their future, and the great value of swimming in the re-adjustment of posture in spinal paraplegics and tetraplegics has already been mentioned. It is now more than 25 years since the Stoke Mandeville Spinal Centre, while under the administration of the former Ministry of Pensions, was provided at my instigation with a therapeutic swimming pool 10 metres long, and hydrotherapy by swimming and training in swimming sport of paraplegics and tetraplegics has played an essential part in their rehabilitation ever since. The first swimming competitions during the national and international games were held there.

The pool has an electric hoist to which a stretcher can be attached to lower tetraplegics during their initial stages of rehabilitation into a bay of the pool, where the physiotherapist,

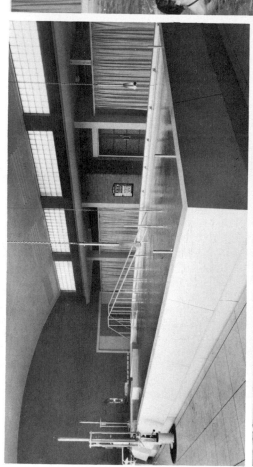

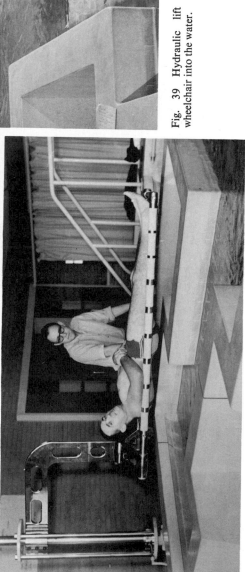

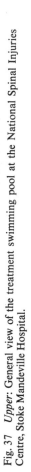

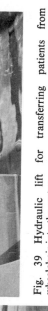

Fig. 39 Hydraulic lift for transferring patients from wheelchair into the water.

Fig. 37 *Upper:* General view of the treatment swimming pool at the National Spinal Injuries Centre, Stoke Mandeville Hospital.

Fig. 38 *Lower:* Hydraulic lift for tetraplegics in the early stages. Note the treatment bay for the physiotherapist.

standing within the encroachment of the bay, can give passive movements to patients with articular or tendineous contractures or marked spasticity in arms and legs. At the same time the tetraplegic can see many of his paralysed fellows already swimming freely which, of course, is a great encouragement to him to do likewise. There is, in addition, another hoist by which patients can be transferred from their wheelchairs and hoisted into the water. However, those more advanced in their rehabilitation are taught to hoist themselves from their chairs into the water with the aid of handles attached to a chain fixed to the ceiling of the pool, or they learn to transfer themselves into the water from a sorbo-rubber mattress situated at the end of the pool as part of the preliminary training for national or international competition in larger pools. The lay-out of this pool is shown in Figs. 37–39. The temperature of the chlorinated water, which is circulating continuously, varies from 82 to 85 °F (28–30° Celsius) and regular bacteriological tests are made to ensure its sterility. With the steadily improving standard of swimming performances of the paralysed during the Stoke Mandeville Games, the competitions have been held in the 6-lane, 25-metre Olympic-size swimming pool of R.A.F. Station, Halton, and for the last 7 years in that of the Stoke Mandeville Sports Stadium for the Paralysed and other Disabled.

As already mentioned, emphasis is laid in spinal paraplegia on *active* hydrotherapy to utilise and mobilise all that is left of the sensory–motor system.

Except for the above-mentioned passive movements for contractures, passive procedures, for instance the so called under-water therapy by douches and other elaborate forms of jets, and other types of passive hydrotherapy which are so popular in European Countries, are not used in the hydrotherapy of the paralysed. The aim of clinical sport through swimming is to encourage the paralysed to improve his performance in contest with himself, and the first thing he learns is to overcome fatigue, that prominent symptom of the early stages of rehabilitation. Moreover, as stressed previously, swimming is invaluable for the development of new movement-patterns of the body which promote postural control in the water.

Training in Hospital

The Conditioning Period

Training starts with the patient lying in the water and at first being supported by the instructor, who places one hand underneath the small of his back and the other under his chin, in order to keep the patient's back and legs raised. In complete lesions, especially those which are spastic, the paralysed part of the body has a tendency to float at an angle varying from 45° in cervical and mid-thoracic lesions to approximately 20° in lower-cord lesions. (Fig. 40). The angle also depends on the height and weight of the patient. Tall individuals will drag their legs further down into the water, while fat individuals will float much more readily than thin ones. In the early stages of training, the higher the lesion the further back the head must be kept to prevent dragging down the legs and to preserve the equilibrium of the body.

The time of adjustment to the water naturally varies according to the level of the spinal cord lesion, age, and whether or not the individual was a skilled swimmer before his spinal cord injury. Those who were skilled swimmers before their paralysis, can adjust themselves to the water in a very short time, sometimes in a few minutes. In fact, one of my former patients who sustained a complete paraplegia below the waist as the result of a fracture dislocation of the spine through falling from a rock into the sea, and hitting another rock during the fall, instantly adjusted himself to his new condition and thus saved his life by swimming breaststroke ashore using his arms only. Another patient—an officer who was thrown into the water when his ship was torpedoed during the Second World War—received his paraplegia from a shell while in the water. He immediately

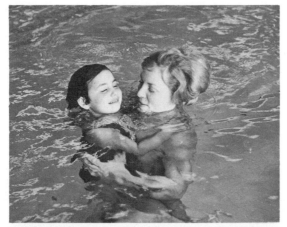

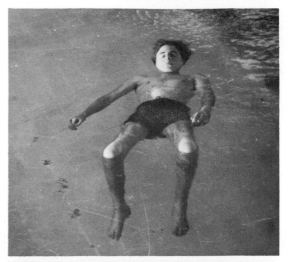

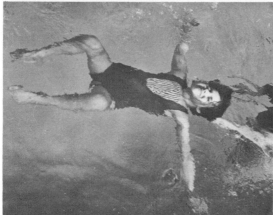

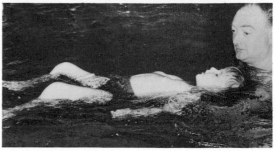

Fig. 40 *Upper*: Paraplegic with mid-thoracic complete paraplegia. Note how the paralysed part of the body floats in the water.

Fig. 41 *Lower*: A 3-year-old paraplegic child being taught to swim.

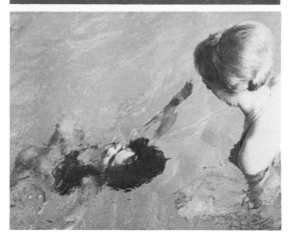

Fig. 42 *Left, top to bottom*: A paraplegic girl clings to her physiotherapist at first but later overcomes her fear and learns to swim.

Fig. 43   Training in back
stroke. Note how the floating
paralysed flexed knees are
extended on adduction of the
arms and extension of the back.

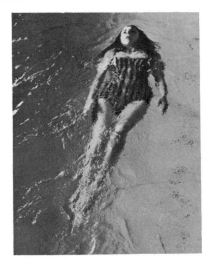 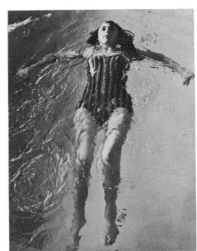

adjusted himself and, using his arms, saved his
life by swimming ashore.

Training in swimming at Stoke Mandeville
has commenced from the age of three and in
older people up to the age of 70. One woman of
61 is worth mentioning: she sustained a complete motor paralysis from the waist down as a
result of polio some years ago and although she
had never swum in her life she took a great
interest in the training and succeeded in becoming a very good and enthusiastic swimmer.

The problem of adjustment of the very young
needs special mention. We have begun to train
children to swim from the age of three. Paralysed children on the whole greatly enjoy swimming lessons and Figure 41 shows a boy of $3\frac{1}{2}$
during his early training; after four months he
was able to take part in a competition for
children. However, some paralysed children—
like the able-bodied of their own age—are
terrified when first lowered into the water and
cling tightly to the necks of their attendants
(Fig. 42). It needs great patience, firmness and
perseverance on the part of the instructor to
overcome this anxiety and at the same time to
teach the paralysed child to swim. The favourite
stroke in the beginning is the back stroke.

Individual Strokes

Backstroke. The first stroke the patient learns
is sculling in the back position, i e. keeping his
hands under water until he has learned to maintain his equilibrium. This is done by alternating
abduction and adduction of the arms. On abduction, the arms are relaxed from the shoulder
joint, the fingers being held in a neutral position
and the forearms slightly flexed. On adduction
of the arms, the forearms are extended, the
wrists being fixed in a neutral position, and the
fingers brought together in order to gain maximum impetus from the stroke. The body is kept
in hyperextension.

Once this basic stroke has been mastered, the
patient is taught the old English back stroke, in
which the arms are brought simultaneously out
of the water over the head, at the same time
maintaining the hyperextension of the spine.
The arms must be relaxed when brought out of
the water. On returning the arms to the body in
adduction, elbow, wrist and fingers are kept in
the same position as outlined previously, and
care should be taken that the arms do not dig
too deeply into the water, as this reduces the
efficiency of the stroke and in mid-thoracic
lesions of spastic type may initiate spasms of
the legs (Fig. 43).

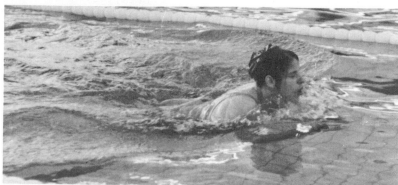

Fig. 44   Breast stroke. Note the extension of the trunk.

Breast stroke. The breast stroke presents different problems. In thoracic lesions, due to paralysis of the extensor muscles of the spine on the one hand and the buoyancy of the hips and legs on the other, the patient either tends to swim in a vertical position which is very difficult because of the maximum resistance which the body offers to the water, or the buoyancy of the paralysed parts of the body tends to topple the upper part of the body from the vertical into the horizontal position, forcing him to swim face downwards in the water. However, with increased training of the latissimus dorsi, trapezius and other shoulder muscles, hyperextension of the spine gradually improves and the patient adjusts himself to a technique which best suits him (Fig. 44). As a result, he will swim two or three strokes face down in the water, then lengthen the stroke and at the same time hyperextend his back and bring his head out of the water. It is important to keep the fingers adducted throughout the stroke to derive maximum impetus from it. Therefore, patients with low cervical lesions (C 8, T 1), although their long extensor and flexors of wrist and fingers are of full power, have a definite disadvantage as compared with lesions below T 2, as the loss of weakness of their intrinsic finger muscles, interossei and lumbricals, prevent them from adducting the fingers. Tetraplegics are also taught to swim face downwards to improve the vital capacity of the lungs, and by the time they leave the Centre they may be able to swim one length of

the 10-metre pool face down. During training, the tetraplegic is supported around the waist and gradually the number of strokes face down is increased before he stops swimming and is turned over on to his back.

Crawl. The crawl presents yet another problem. As the legs in complete lesions cannot be used to stabilize the body, it will rotate with each stroke of the arm. This can be overcome in the back crawl to a certain extent by a sculling action with the arm which is in the water. However, by achieving greater skill the sculling action can be abandoned. The problem of rotation exists also for the front crawl. It is known that able-bodied swimmers also rotate their bodies in the water, but this is less pronounced because rotation of the hips and pelvis can be prevented by the active movements of the legs. In paraplegics and tetraplegics, the whole trunk and pelvis will rotate, as the paralyzed legs cannot counteract the rotation of the pelvis. This is particularly conspicuous in tetraplegics, due to the paralysis of most of the trunk muscles. Only in exceptional cases of tetraplegia at the level of C 7/8 will the patient be able to use the crawl (Fig. 45).

Butterfly stroke. This has only recently been introduced into the swimming training of paraplegics and has become part of the Stoke Mandeville Games, as have free-style competitions.

Team water sports, such as medley, are always among the competitions of the Games. Water-polo has also been practised but has not yet developed as a team competition due to lack of proper facilities.

Competition Training in Swimming

As soon as the individual's progress is sufficiently advanced and he shows an interest in training for participation in the Stoke Mandeville Games and other competitions, a training schedule should be organised for him which includes the method of interval training. As our national and international sports meetings are held between June and August, the training schedule can be divided into three periods:

Preliminary Training
This should take place between August and October and include improving experience gained in the various swimming strokes at medium speed, and learning to start and turn. During this period, field events and track training can also be used to build up muscular strength and the adjustment potentials of the cardiovascular and respiratory systems.

Pre-competition Training
This should take place between October and January. During this period, competitors concentrate on increasing speed gradually in relation to the distance at which they intend to compete. Moreover, practice in starting and turning is intensified to minimise loss of time. Training in additional sports is cut down during this period.

Controlled Interval Training
This training, which takes place between January and June, consists of concentration on speed work over short distances, progressive increase of speed and distance and overcoming fatigue by shortening the length of recovery intervals.

Rules

The rules for all swimming competitions are adapted from the rules of the International Amateur Swimming Association (FINA), naturally with amendments and modifications necessary for the paralysed. The competitors are divided into classes: three types of cervical motor lesion—two

Fig. 45 Paraplegic patient in back crawl exercises.

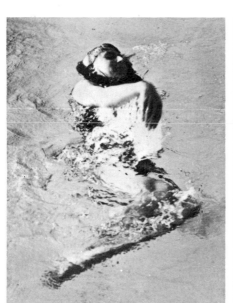
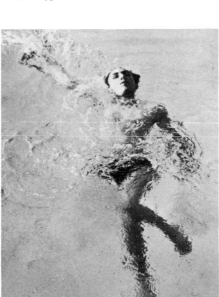

types of thoracic lesions—three types of distal thorax and lumbar lesions limited to the lower limbs.

1. *Cervical Level*

Class 1a. All cervical lesions with complete paralysis of the triceps or very weak function of that muscle—i e. up to power 3 of the M R C testing points system.

Class 1b. All cervical lesions with preservation of a normal or subnormal triceps and good extension of the wrist (power 4-5 M R C testing points system)

Class 1c, which also includes the first thoracic segments (T 1), are those with normal function of the triceps, long extensors and flexors of wrist and fingers but with paralysis or great weakness of the intrinsic muscles of the fingers, interossei, lumbricals and thumb muscles. As mentioned before, due to the paralysis of these muscles proper adduction of the fingers is not possible which decreases significantly the efficiency of the stroke.

2. *Thoracic Level*

Class 2. Lesions below T 1 to T 5 inclusive.

Class 3. Lesions below T 5 to T 10 inclusive.

3. *Lower Thoracic—and Lumbar Level*

Class 4. Lesions below T 10 to L 3 inclusive.

Class 5. Lesions below L 3 to L 5 inclusive.

Class 6. Lesions below L 5. These competitors have the great advantage of full extension of hips and legs and good dorsi- and plantar flexion of feet and toes.

Competitors with higher lesions are allowed to take part in contests with those having lower lesions, if they feel competent to do so and provided there is no objection from a medical or trainer's point of view. Hereunder is a summary of some of the essential details of the rules:

The Pool and Swimming Course

The course for paralysed swimmers at the Stoke Mandeville Games shall be not less than 25 metres in length, and at least six lanes each 2.25 metres wide shall be provided on the surface of the water. When the finishing point is not at the end of the swimming pool, a pole or other rigid line shall be provided.

Before the start, the starter must describe to the contestants the course of the competition, the turning and finishing points and their correct lanes previously agreed by the judges and referees. After two false starts a warning is given that the race will proceed at the third

attempt irrespective of further infringements. The starter shall then disqualify any offending competitor at the third start whether he was a previous offender or not. To be eligible for the final event, the competitor must have competed in the preliminary heats. The six fastest times qualify for the final. Dead-heaters in the preliminary heats are entitled to swim in the finals.

Jostling or swimming across and obstructing another competitor so as to impede his progress disqualifies the offender, but a swimmer who has been fouled is allowed to compete in the next heat or final. If a foul has occurred in a final the judges may order a re-swim.

The rules for starting and swimming differ according to the type of stroke. The start in all races for the paralysed is made with the competitors already in the water.

Swimming Strokes

Only swimmers in Class C 5 and 6 may use their legs.

Back stroke: the competitors line up in the water facing the starting end of the pool, with both hands resting on the edge or rail or starting grips (Fig. 46). The feet, including the toes, shall be under the surface of the water. Standing in or on the gutter or bending the toes over the lip of the gutter is not allowed. At the signal for starting, they push off with their hands, and at the height of the push hyperextend the back while throwing their arms back into the water (Fig. 46) and continuing to swim on their backs throughout the race. Any competitor leaving the back position before his head or foremost hand or arm has touched the turn or finishing point, is disqualified. The turn and finish in the back stroke contest are a one-hand touch, in accordance with international rules.

Breast stroke: the competitors line up in the water facing the pool, holding the rail or end of the back or other starting place with at least one hand (Fig. 47). After the signal to start has been given one asymmetric stroke is permitted to allow the swimmer to attain the breast stroke

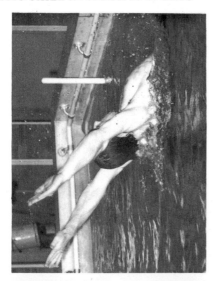

Fig. 46   Start of back stroke race

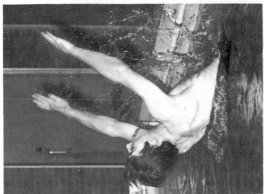

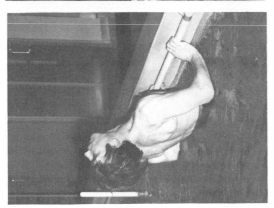

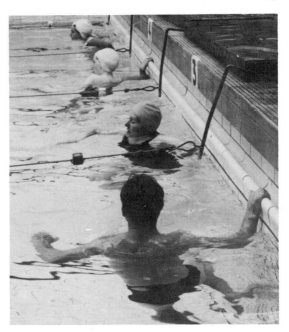

Fig. 47   Start of breast stroke race.

position. (In Classes 1a and 1b the decision for disqualification will rest with the referee and representative of the I S M G Technical Committee.)

All movements of legs and arms shall be simultaneous and in the same horizontal plane without alternating movement. In the leg-kick the feet must be turned outwards in the backward movement. The Dolphin kick is not allowed. Competitors in Classes 5 and 6 must conform to the above or allow their legs to drag.

Both hands shall be pushed forward together from the breast on or under the surface of the water and brought back simultaneously and symmetrically with lateral extension.

The body shall be kept on the breast and when touching at the turn, or finish of a race, the touch shall be made with both hands simultaneously on the same level. (In Classes 1a and 1b any infringement of this will be dealt with by the referee and a member of the ISMGF Commmittee.)

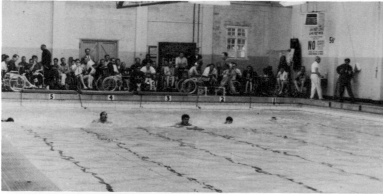

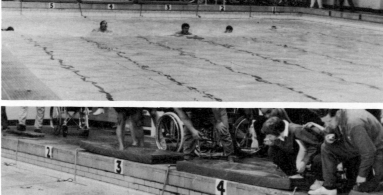

Fig. 48   Start and finish of a breast stroke race during the Stoke Mandeville Games.

The competitor is prohibited from swimming under the surface of the water except one complete arm stroke after start and turn, and may take one stroke to assist him to return promptly to the surface. Either a complete or incomplete movement of the arms shall be considered as one stroke (Fig. 48).

When a swimmer, after start or turn, begins the second stroke, one part of the head shall always break the surface of the water (if there is any doubt of this infringement for medical reasons, a member of the I S M G F Committee will be consulted).

Butterfly Stroke: both arms must be brought forward together over the water and brought backward simultaneously. The body must be kept perfectly on the breast and both shoulders in line with the surface of the water from the be-

ginning of the first arm stroke, after starting and on the turn.

Touching on the turn or on finishing the race must be made with both hands simultaneously on the same level and with the shoulders in the horizontal position. The touch may be made at above or below the water level.

Freestyle front swimming: competitors can use the crawl. They line up in the water facing down the pool, as in breast stroke, holding with at least one hand on the rail. At the starting signal, they push off and swim in the prone position throughout the race. In turning, competitors may touch the end of the course with any part of the body, but in finishing, the touch must be made with at least one hand.

In freestyle swimming, which is included in the medley and relay competitions, the competitors line up in the water holding the rails or side of the bath or other starting place. They may swim in any style other than breast, back stroke or butterfly, and the rules relating specifically to breast stroke or back stroke shall not apply.

The following are the events and distances which can be competed for by swimmers in the Paraplegic Games:

TABLE 7. Swimming Events

Classes 1a, b & c	25 m	Breast Back Freestyle
Class 2	25 m	Breast Back Freestyle Butterfly
Classes 3 & 4	50 m	Breast Back Freestyle
	25 m	Butterfly
Class 5	100 m	Breast Back Freestyle
	50 m	Butterfly
Class 6	50 m	Butterfly
	100 m	Breast Back Freestyle Butterfly
Classes 2 & 3	3×25 m	Ind. Medley
Classes 4, 5 & 6	3×50 m	Ind. Medley

3-Person Medley Relay (3×50 m): one Class 2, one Class 3 & one Class 4
3-Person Medley Relay (3×100 m): Open Class
4-Person Medley Relay (4×100 m): Open Class
4-Person Freestyle Relay (4×50 m): one Class 1, one Class 2, one Class 3 & one Class 4, 5 & 6.
Individual Medley: Classes 2 & 3—3×25 m; Classes 4, 5 & 6—3×50 m.

Records

World records are recognised for both sexes in the above events under the supervision of officials appointed or approved by the I S M G F Committee and made in a scratch competition on an individual race against time, held in public.

Tables 8–10 list the records achieved in recent years during the I S M G swimming competitions by male and female competitors in the various classes. For comparison Table 11 gives the records of able-bodied swimmers in 100-metre competions.

In relays, the first swimmer may attempt to break an existing world or national record if he, his coach or manager specifically request that this performance be treated as a record attempt.

The master copy of world records is kept at the Stoke Mandeville Stadium, and all such records must be ratified by the I S M G F Committee

Sub-Aqua Diving

This adventure sport, using snorkel and aqua-lung, has become increasingly popular amongst the able-bodied, but in recent years it has been proved that paralysed people can also be trained in this sport and can enjoy it, especially those who had practised it before they became paralysed. A former patient of Stoke Mandeville National Spinal Injuries Centre, Nicholas Flemming, an experienced sub-aqua diver, sustained a traumatic complete paraplegia below the mid-thoracic region. This did not prevent him, after rehabilitation, from returning to his former job at the National Institute of Oceanography and taking up sub-aqua swimming again and, indeed, teaching it to other paraplegics. Figures 49–51 (p. 76) show him demonstrating underwater swimming with his aqua-lung equipment and snorkel in the Stoke Mandeville Sports Stadium. A short time ago, he held a successful training course in this sport at Haifa University in Israel. From all his experiences, Flemming came to the conclusion that paraplegics up to T 5 level can be trained to dive in a pool and in the open sea provided certain precautions and restrictions are observed. Paraplegics above T 5 may also be trained to use aqua-lung equipment

CLASS	STYLE	1970		RECORD	
		MEN	WOMEN	MEN	WOMEN
1a Upper cervical: triceps up to and inc. Grade 3 MRC Scale	Breast Back F/style	70·4 sec 74·8 sec 115·7 sec	150·8 sec 50·5 sec 70·0 sec	60·4 sec 36·0 sec 33·5 sec	46·5 sec 38·5 sec 38·9 sec
1b Lower cervical: good triceps, wrist ext. & flex. finger flex. & ext. below Grade 3	Breast Back F/style	35·0 sec 29·4 sec 25·2 sec	39·6 sec 37·5 sec 34·4 sec	30·2 sec 25·5 sec	39·6 sec 37·5 sec 34·4 sec
1c* Lower cervical: good triceps, strong finger flex & ext. to power 4; no interossei or lumbrical	Breast Back F/style			32·1 sec 30·2 sec 26·1 sec	36·1 sec 33·2 sec 28·6 sec
2 Below T 1 to T 5 inc. no balance when sitting	Breast Back F/style	28·0 sec 29·6 sec 27·5 sec	37·9 sec 35·8 sec 33·0 sec	25·5 sec 23·9 sec 18·7 sec	26·9 sec 26·8 sec 20·4 sec

TABLE 8. Records achieved at 25-metre Swimming in Classes 1a, 1b, 1c and 2.

* New class, introduced in 1974.

CLASS	STYLE	1970		RECORD	
		MEN	WOMEN	MEN	WOMEN
3 *T 6 to* *T 10*	Breast Back F/Style	53·6 sec 52·6 sec 47·2 sec	1 min 20·5 sec 1 min 13·5 sec 1 min 20·0 sec	48·9 sec 42·2 sec 37·3 sec	56·6 sec 49·0 sec 47·0 sec
4 *T 11 to* *L 3*	Breast Back F/Style	55·0 sec 45·4 sec 43·6 sec	60·0 sec 56·2 sec 47·8 sec	46·3 sec 41·2 sec 35·3 sec	55·5 sec 46·6 sec 35·8 sec

TABLE 9. Records achieved at 50-metre Swimming in Classes 3 and 4.

in a swimming pool, but as a rule should be excluded from diving in the sea because of the increased risk. The diving training for paraplegics and other disabled should always be done under the closest supervision: careful selection of pupils is imperative, and the instructor should be aware of the paraplegic's limitations. They should undergo a detailed medical examination with special reference to possible side effects arising from their physical defect. Flemming is right to draw attention to deficiencies of the respiratory and cardiovascular systems (among others) and the dangers of 'bends' as a result of rapid decompression. I would, therefore, question the

TABLE 10. Records achieved at 100-metre Swimming in Classes 5 and 6.

CLASS	STYLE	1970		RECORD	
		MEN	WOMEN	MEN	WOMEN
5	Breast	2 min 1·3 sec	2 min 15·0 sec	1 min 37·4 sec	1 min 42·8 sec
	Back			1 min 18.9 sec	1 min 23·5 sec
	F/Style	1 min 52·6 sec	1 min 36·8 sec	1 min 12·3 sec	1 min 19·0 sec
6	Breast	1 min 45·1 sec		1 min 40·0 sec	1 min 45·1 sec
	Back			1 min 23·8 sec	1 min 21·5 sec
	F/Style	1 min 14·7 sec	1 min 13·4 sec	1 min 10·4 sec	1 min 12·4 sec

STYLE	WORLD		BRITISH NATIONAL	
	MEN	WOMEN	MEN	WOMEN
Breast	1 min 04·02 sec	1 min 13·58 sec	1 min 05·74 sec	1 min 15·82 sec
Back	56·3 sec	1 min 04·43 sec	1 min 00·3 sec	1 min 08·57 sec
F/Style	51·22 sec	57·71 sec	53·4 sec	1 min 00·5 sec
Butterfly	54·27 sec	1 min 02·31 sec	58·13 sec	1 min 05·96 sec
	ENGLISH SHORT COURSE		1973 ASA CHAMPIONSHIPS	
	MEN	WOMEN	MEN	WOMEN
Breast	1 min 08·4 sec	1 min 15·1 sec	1 min 07·88 sec	1 min 17·93 sec
Back	1 min 00·7 sec	1 min 08·4 sec	1 min 00·76 sec	1 min 09·98 sec
F/Style	53·9 sec	1 min 00·5 sec	54·62 sec	1 min 00·71 sec
Butterfly	57·4 sec	1 min 07·0 sec	58·9 sec	1 min 06·26 sec

TABLE 11. Able-bodied 100 metres swimming records.

rationale for including paraplegics at T 5/6 level in the training to dive in the open sea in view of the unstable vasomotor control resulting from the damage to the splanchnic nerves at that level. Frankel (1975) has emphasized the dangers of cardio-vascular complication caused by sub-aqua diving in depths below 50 metres. Flemming's suggestion that the disabled diver after his intial training should join a diving club or school with qualified instructors is sound, as is his advice that no disabled diver should dive with other disabled or alone. He should dive with two able-bodied experienced divers, who remain close to the disabled diver in the water, and know his limitations. In the sea, the paralysed diver should avoid coral reefs and rocks to prevent abrasions; he should avoid diving in strong winds and high waves and never go inside caves or wrecks. Training sessions in sub-aqua diving are given at the Stoke Mandeville Stadium swimming pool to paraplegics with distal injuries of the spinal cord by Mr Peter Pauley, an experienced coach in this adventure sport.

There will always be exceptions to the rules and among the spinal injured and other disabled there are adventurous people just as there are among the able-bodied. As a glaring example of re-adjustment, one of my former tetraplegic

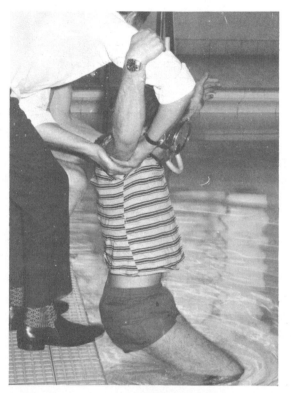

patients may be mentioned, an expert skin diver before his accident when he sustained a complete tetraplegia below the C 5/6 segments, the only well functioning muscles of the upper limbs being the deltoid and biceps. After being retrained at Stoke Mandeville, he continued swimming on his return to Kenya, and, in due course, took up underwater swimming in spite of his wife's, friends' and doctor's misgivings, using two snorkels, one built into the mask as an air intake through the nose and an ordinary snorkel held in the mouth to expel waste air. This system worked well, with the air in the mask providing a buoyant 'pillow' for his head. He also proceeded to use an aqua-lung which needed more organisation, including an experienced diver with a second aqua-lung, to tow him along at the bottom of the sea, in addition to a third diver with underwater camera equipment to record the proceedings and to supply documentary proof. He was lowered over the side of the boat to sink slowly into 15 feet of water. He wrote: "Undersea diving was always a passion of mine, so to see again the ripple shadows on the coral beds and all the teeming varieties of brilliant fish was a sensation that can be imagined. Breathing was perfectly normal, and apart from a slight tendency to rise by the tail and sink by the head I felt absolutely comfortable. I find that underwater movement is much freer. My limited neck and shoulder wriggle exerts more purchase below than on the surface. The next

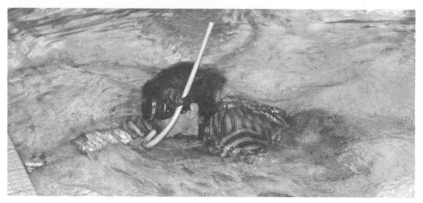

Fig. 49 *Upper*: Sub-aqua swimming—lowering a paraplegic swimmer into the water.

Fig. 50 Snorkel swimming.

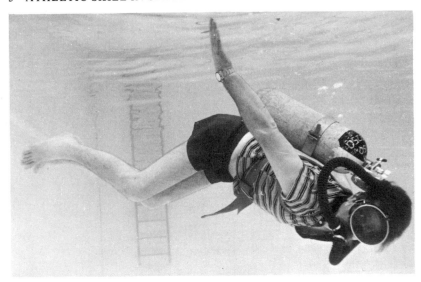

Fig. 51 Sub-aqua swimming with aqualung.

attempt was as successful, and although I have so far only reached 20 feet down, I am currently designing a pair of strap-on elbow fins for stronger swimming, so who knows?"

FIELD EVENTS

Field events, including distance and precision javelin throwing, shot put, discus and club throwing have been practised in the S M G from an early date. As already pointed out, field events have proved invaluable for restoring and improving the equilibrium of the paralysed as well as the power of the muscles of trunk and upper limbs. These sports are conducted in accordance with the international athletic rules of the able-bodied adapted for wheelchair athletes. All field events are carried out with the competitor sitting in his wheelchair. In all field events, competitors are divided according to their physical deficit, as there is no doubt that the loss of the abdominals and lower trunk muscles produces an increased handicap. The classes in operation in field events are the same as those described for swimming competitions, with the exception that Class 6 is excluded.

General Rules for all Field Events

Each class is allocated its own throwing area and all the throwing competitions for that particular class are carried out in that area. The competitors, if they so desire, may throw all their implements one after the other if this has been noted on the entry form.

The throwing area consists of a throwing circle enclosed by a raised metal band which prevents the wheels of the competitor's chair from going over the front line of the circle, but allows clearance of the foot plates.

The circle has an inside diameter of 2.15 m. The throwing sector is marked by radial lines 5 cm wide which form an angle of 65° from the centre of the circle. The wheels of the chair must be behind the stop board of the circle; only the foot rest may be over but not touching the metal board.

Wheelchairs are, if possible, anchored by apparatus approved by the I S M G Committee. If such apparatus is not available, officials may permit the chair to be held but the holding person must be entirely within the circle or the throw will be judged a foul throw; neither the holder, the coach nor anyone else may assist the competitor, and any infringement may result in the disqualification of the competitor.

The measurement of each throw shall be made from the nearest mark made by the fall of the point of the javelin or discus, shot or club to the inside circumference of the circle, along a line from the mark made by the implement to the centre of the circle. In each sector the record throw in each event and for each class throwing in that sector shall be marked as follows:

Record Javelin Throw	— Yellow Marker
Record Discus Throw	— Blue Marker
Record Club Throw	— Red Marker
Record Shot Put	— White Marker

Records of distances shall be indicated on a board.

A soft cushion of maximum thickness 10 cm (4 in), the size of the chair seat, may be used.

No hard board is allowed under the cushion.

Competitors have to remain seated in their chairs and their feet remain on the foot rest until the throw is completed. A competitor may be allowed at the conclusion of his throw and as continuation of the throw, to roll his buttock on the throwing side from the cushion, but this must not constitute a definite lift in the chair during the throw. Also as a continuation of the throw the foot on the throwing side may be allowed to come off the footrest but not touch the ground.

Restraining straps round the legs for spasm are permitted if authorised and entered on the medical identity card by a member of the I S M G medical team.

All throws to be valid must fall within the inner edge of the lines marking the sector.

In Classes 1a–c throws in all events will be considered good throws if delivered with the competitor facing the throwing area.

If a competitor leaves from the front of the circle after his throw, his last throw will be declared a foul.

If a competitor's feet or footrest touch the ground or metal band before the throw is completed it will be declared a foul throw. Competitors are forbidden to use any additions or implements fixed to the chair to give them an unfair advantage.

Preliminary Training

The preliminary training in all field events, which takes place between September and March, is not confined to the techniques of the individual events but is directed to the development of concentration and the building-up of general strength, fitness and speed (perfection depends greatly on speed×strength) as well as mobilization of shoulder and elbow joints. Table tennis, ball games and resistance exercises, graduated weight training and, whenever possible, rope climbing are useful methods to achieve this aim. In the actual training for individual events, emphasis is laid on the posture of the arms in relation to the trunk, and smoothness of performance rather than vigour. Those athletes who have already taken part in competitions may use this period for correcting faults and concentrating on modifications or alterations to their own technique.

Pre-Competition Training

In the period between March and May, strength, smoothness and endurance of the acquired techniques in the various events have to be developed and the whole tempo of training increased. Weight training and general exercise must not be neglected at this stage. Competitions at this stage are also important.

Competition Training

In the competition season, the acquired techniques should be altered basically and the amount of hard throwing cut down to prevent overstrain of shoulder and elbow. Resistance and warming-up exercises can be helpful during this period. One or two days' rest before competition should be allowed following hard training.

Techniques and Rules in specific Field Events

Distance Javelin

The javelin should be made of metal or solid wood with a metal point and is the women's Olympic type model which conforms to the following specification:

Min. length	2·20 m (7 ft 2·614 in)
Dist. from point to centre of gravity	min 80 cm (2 ft 7·496 in) max 95 cm (3 ft 1·401 in)
Min. Weight	600 g (1 lb 5·163 oz)

The cord grip situated about the centre of gravity should be 15.0 cm (5.85 in) wide and its circumference at either end should not exceed the circumference of the javelin shaft by more

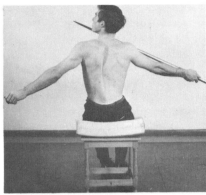

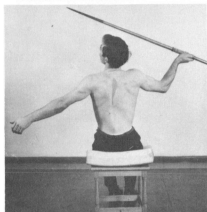

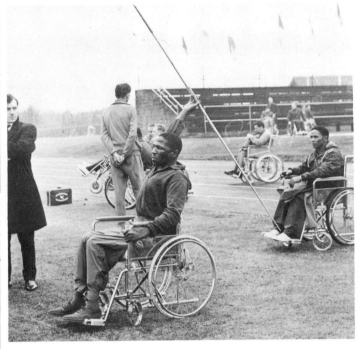

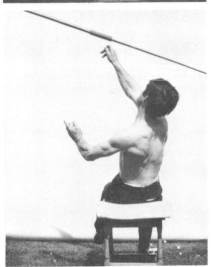

Fig. 52 *Left*: Training in javelin throwing.

Fig. 53 *Above*: South African athletes in javelin throwing competition.

than 2.5 cm (1 in). Thongs, notches and indentations of any kind on the shaft are not allowed.

During the contest, the javelin is held by the cord grip with one hand only and the throw must be made from behind the arc and fall into the sector, the point striking before the shaft. Delivery of the javelin must be made over the shoulder or upper part of the throwing arm and it must not be slung or hurled. The competitor's last contact with the javelin during the release must be the cord grip. During the competition, three throws are allowed, the three to six best competitors being allowed a further three throws. Each finalist will be credited with the best of his six throws. If there is a tie, the second best performance will decide the winner.

Foul throws are caused by the following offences:

1. The javelin falling on or outside the lines marking the sector.
2. The point of the javelin not striking the ground first.
3. The competitor not holding the javelin by the cord grip.

The measurement of the throw is made from the nearest edge of the first mark made by the javelin to the inside circumference of the arc (along a line from the mark made by the javelin to the centre of the circle). All measurements are

TABLE 12. Records achieved in Javelin.

CLASS	1970		RECORD	
	MEN	WOMEN	MEN	WOMEN
2	18·05 m	8·31 m	20·97 m	11·56 m
3	19·50 m	12·88 m	24·83 m	13·88 m
4	25·05 m	14·17 m	25·53 m	14·17 m
5	25·59 m	14·82 m	31·60 m	18·50 m

	MEN	WOMEN
World Record (Able-bodied)	94·08 m	66·10 m
UK Record (Able-Bodied)	84·92 m	55·66 m
AAA Standard (Senior) Class 1	68·00 m	0306
Class 2	64·00 m	
Class 3	56·00 m	

made with a certified steel tape (Figs. 52 & 53). From Table 12 it will be seen that there is an increasing standard in both men's and women's competitions.

Precision Javelin Throwing

This sport is specifically designed for wheelchair athletes and, like darts, requires discriminate movements of the shoulder and arm muscles, unlike the powerful thrust achieved by the forceful action of trunk, shoulder and arm muscles in distance javelin throwing. The type of javelin and faults in throwing, are the same as described in distance javelin throwing.

The competitor in the precision javelin throwing contest is allowed six throws, the five best to count. The target (Fig. 54), has a diameter of 3 m (9 ft 10.25 in) and consists of 8 rings of 20 cm approximately. Ring 1=2 points, progressing to Ring 8=16 points. Hitting the line of a circle counts as the number above. Male competitors throw from a distance of 10 metres (32 ft 9.666 in) and females from 7 metres (22 ft 11.5 in) measured from the centre of the target.

Figure 54 compares the postural differences between precision and distance javelin throwing.

Shot Put

The shot, being a solid sphere made of iron or brass, weighs 4 kg for male and 3 kg for female competitors and 2 kg for male and female competitors of Classes 1a, b & c. The minimum diameter is 9.5 cm (3.741 in), and the maximum 11 cm (4.330 in).

A legal shot put is made from the shoulder with one hand only. At the commencement of the put the shot shall touch or be in close proximity to the chin and the hand shall not be dropped below this position during the action of putting. The shot must not be brought behind the line of the shoulders (Fig. 56). Before the

TABLE 13. Records achieved in Shot Put.

CLASS	1970		RECORD	
	MEN	WOMEN	MEN	WOMEN
2	7·20 m	3·93 m	7·90 m	4·88 m
3	7·30 m	5·10 m	9·23 m	6·31 m
4	7·98 m	6·59 m	8·57 m	6·59 m
5	8·85 m	6·82 m	10·48 m	7·17 m

	MEN	WOMEN
World Record (Able-bodied)	21·82 m	21·20 m
UK Record (Able-bodied)	21·37 m	16·31 m
AAA Standard (Senior) Class 1	17·00 m	
Class 2	16·00 m	
Class 3	14·00 m	

Fig. 54   *Left*: Precision javelin throwing.

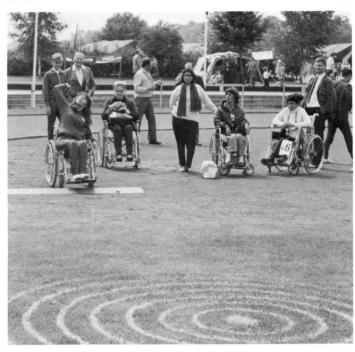

Fig. 55   *Below*: Precision (*left*) and distance javelin throwing: difference in posture.

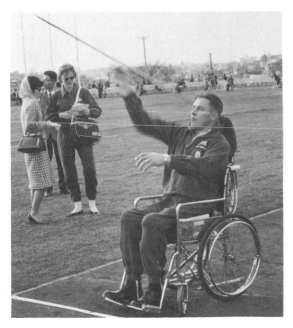

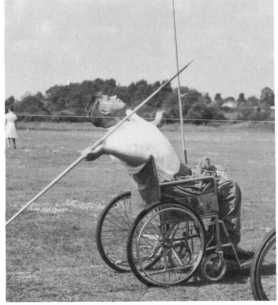

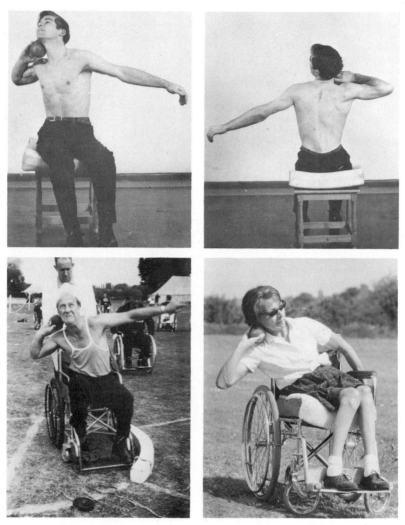

Fig. 56   Shot put training.

Fig. 57   Shot put contestants.

shot the wheelchair shall be firmly secured because for every pound effort which pushes the shot forward there is an equal push through the back of the chair to the ground which will tip the chair to some extent and thus lessen the efficiency of the throw. The chair should be at 45° right to the direction of the throw, while the left hand, in the case of a right-hander, acting as a purchase grips the armrest of the chair. The use of harness or any mechanical device attached to the hand or arm is not permitted. Taping the wrist, palm or back of the hand is allowed, provided that not more than two joining fingers are taped. During the competition, three puts are allowed, the three to six best competitors being allowed a further three puts. Each finalist will be credited with the best of his six shot puts. If there is a tie the second best performance will decide the winner; if there is again a tie the third best. Foul puts are those which:

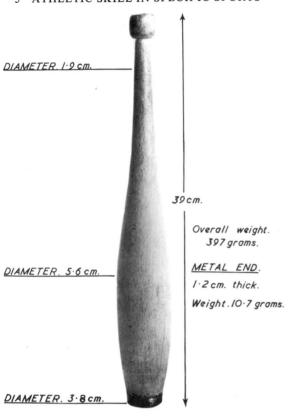

DIAMETER. 1·9 cm.

39 cm.

Overall weight.
397 grams.

METAL END.
1·2 cm. thick.
Weight. 10·7 grams.

DIAMETER. 5·6 cm.

DIAMETER. 3·8 cm.

Fig. 58 The throwing club.

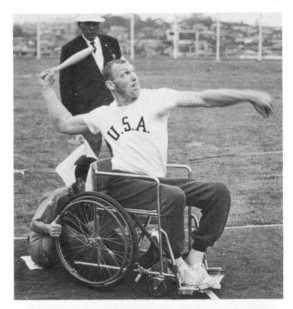

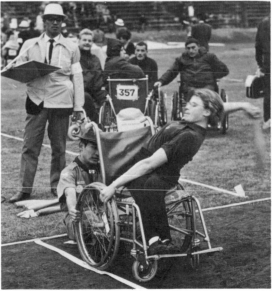

Fig. 59 Club throwing competitions during the Games.

(a) do not conform to the definition of a legal put, and

(b) cause the shot to fall on or outside the lines marking the sector.

Fig. 57 shows shot put contests, Table 13 the records achieved.

Club Throwing

The club takes the place of the javelin in Classes 1a and 1b.

The throwing club is made from beech wood, and the details of its shape and measurements are shown in Fig. 58. The throw is carried out from behind a line, and care is taken that the chair is clear of the line and the footrest or chair clear of the ground. The club is thrown like the javelin by a free-style throw. If the club breaks during the release or in the air in a correct

TABLE 14. Records achieved at Throwing the Club.

CLASS	1975	
	MEN	WOMEN
1a	25·13 m	13·41 m
1b	30·61 m	14·46 m

throw, it is not counted as a throw. If the club breaks on contact with the ground, the throw is measured, provided the throw was made in accordance with the rules and no substitute throw is allowed. During the competition, three throws are allowed, the three to six best competitors being allowed a further three throws. Each competitor will be credited with the best of his throws. If there is a tie the second best performance will decide the winner (Fig. 59). Foul throws occur when:

(a) the competitor touches with his chair over the line;

(b) the competitor throws a club which does not conform to the regular specifications;

(c) the competitor does not remain seated in the chair for the throw;

(d) any of the offences mentioned in the general rules and for the javelin contest are committed.

Discus

This sport requires particularly intensive training, for it not only demands great power in the swinging movement of the throwing arm and shoulder, but also appropriate associated movements of the opposite upper limb as well as swinging movements of the trunk from one direction to another. Discus throwing is the field sport in which the athlete will, in the course of training, develop his own favourite throwing technique (Fig. 60).

The discus consists of a wood (or other suitable material) body to which a smooth metal rim is attached, with metal plates set flush into the sides of the body and situated in the exact centre of the discus in order to obtain the correct weight. Each side of the discus must be identical and without projecting points, sharp edges or indentations. The sides should taper in a straight line from the beginning of the curve of the rim to a circle which is a distance of 2.5 cm (1 in) from the centre of the discus. The weight should be 1 kg. The discus must be thrown from the circle and must fall within the sector previously marked. During the competition, three

TABLE 15. Records achieved in Discus.

CLASS	1970		RECORD	
	MEN	WOMEN	MEN	WOMEN
2	20·32 m	9·88 m	22·07 m	14·99 m
3	22·25 m	14·13 m	26·27 m	16·58 m
4	25·55 m	16·61 m	29·91 m	17·05 m
5	28·42 m	21·25 m	37·80 m	24·97 m

	MEN	WOMEN
World Record (Able-bodied)	68·40 m	69·48 m
UK Record (Able-bodied)	64·92 m	58·02 m
AAA Standard (Senior) Class 1	50·00 m	
Class 2	47·00 m	
Class 3	43·00 m	

throws are allowed, the three to six best competitors being allowed a further three throws. Each finalist will be credited with the best of all his throws (Fig. 61; Table 15). If there is a tie, the second best performance will decide the winner, and if there is again a tie the third best.

The same penalties apply to fouls as in the general rules.

TABLE TENNIS

Throughout the years, this sport has gained increasing popularity among both paraplegics and tetraplegics, and today it plays a major part in the national games of most countries, as well as in the I S M G. During hospital treatment, table

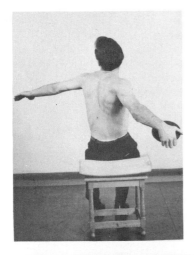
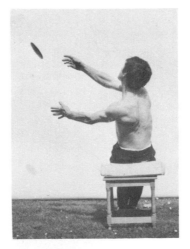
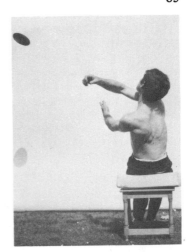

Fig. 60 *Above*: Technique of throwing the discus.

Fig. 61 *Left*: A discus competition.

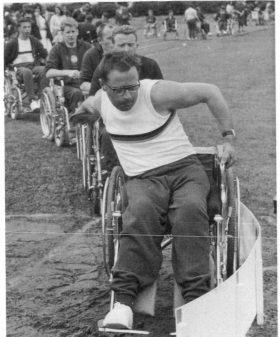

sions, it greatly helps to restore the equilibrium of the paralysed and to promote concentration and activity of mind. Moreover, it also serves as an ideal recreational pastime to overcome boredom in hospital, especially in the wintertime and at weekends. Furthermore, table tennis is a game which can, without great difficulty, be continued at home after the paraplegic is discharged from hospital, and he can compete with members of his family or friends and use this sport as physical exercise and recreational activity.

A basic difference between normal table tennis technique and that of the paralysed player, is that the paraplegic uses his free arm to hold on to his chair to stabilize himself or to hold on to the wheel of his chair to manoeuvre the chair during the game, while the able-bodied player uses his free arm as a counterbalance, as he does in foil fencing. Some tetraplegics may anchor their free arm around the handle of the chair for better support.

Training

In the early stages, training is directed to acquir-

tennis is employed as an invaluable remedial exercises, in addition to the conventional methods of physiotherapy. For, by creating a variety of situations that demand quick deci-

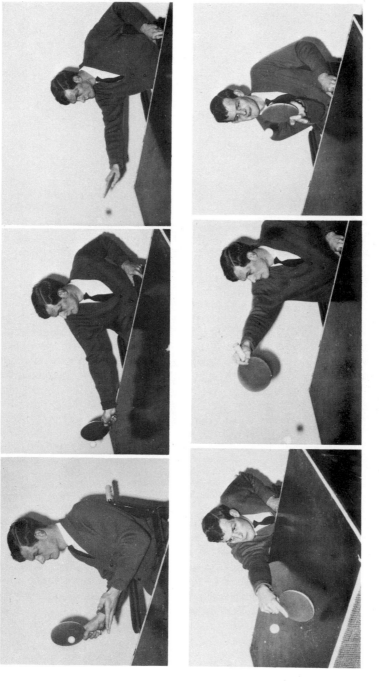
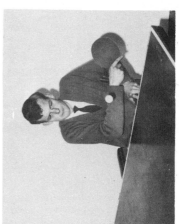

Fig. 62   Serving and volleying techniques in table tennis.

Fig. 63   Lady Susan Masham playing a table tennis match.

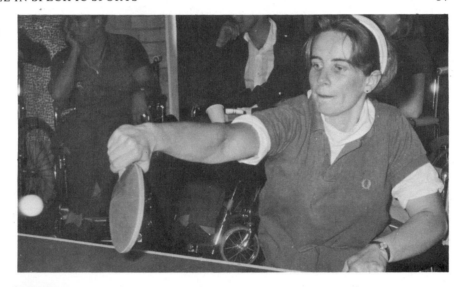

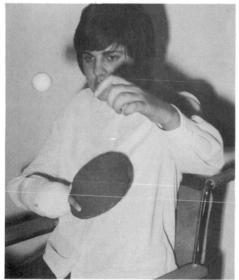

Fig. 64   Ruth Brookes, complete tetraplegic, during a table tennis match. The bat is fixed onto her hand as all her fingers are paralysed.

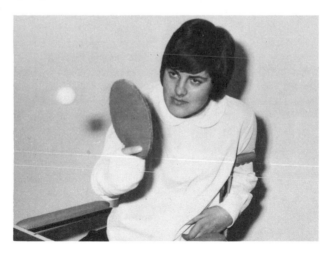

ing complete mastery of gripping the table tennis bat and of the basic strokes. The correct grip must be exercised from the start, for if it is neglected, the player may acquire an awkward style which will make both good service and return strokes difficult, and even impossible. In the orthodox grip, thumb and forefinger will grip the bat from either side, while the other fingers grip the handle. This grip facilitates forehand and backhand play (Fig. 62). A modification is to hold the bat with the thumb only, while the forefinger supports the other fingers in holding the handle. This grip may give greater momentum in backhand serving (Fig. 63). An alternative to the orthodox hold was introduced by the Japanese, the 'pen-hold' style, where the handle of the bat is held as for a pen, i e. between fore and middle fingers. This is, of course, an easy and more natural style for the Japanese, who from early childhood are accustomed to holding chopsticks. However, for people in wheelchairs it is a style which is as a rule very difficult to adopt.

Two types of service are taught in the beginning: Top Spin and Back Spin, to which later on Side Spin is added. In order to build up the rally, it is necessary to keep the ball in play, and to achieve this, the Push Stroke is taught in both backhand and forehand version, the backhand Push Stroke being the more commonly used. Amongst the attacking strokes which follow the simple strokes in training, the Top Spin Drive, in which the forefinger plays a very important part by being moved up the blade of the bat to exert pressure for controlling speed, is the most important one to master. A variation of this stroke is the slow Top Spin, which, however, can be easily counter-hit by the defending player. Furthermore, backhand and forehand defence have to be included and exercised in training. Finally, all the variations of the above strokes, eg. half volley and drop shots, have to be mastered to achieve a high degree of skill at table tennis.

Special mention must be made of the participation of tetraplegics in table tennis. Owing to the paralysis of their finger and thumb muscles in lesions below C 6 and C 7 levels, they are unable to hold the bat unassisted. However, a considerable number are able to play table tennis well, so long as the deltoid, biceps and triceps muscles are functioning, provided, as mentioned before, the table tennis bat is fastened to the hand and fingers in the orthodox hold by means of a bandage (Fig. 64).

Even if the triceps is paralysed, it is still possible for tetraplegics of Classes 1a & b to play table tennis. Tetraplegics at these levels cannot serve from the flat hand and are allowed, therefore, to place the ball between the top of the thumb and the forefinger and throw it upwards to serve. The skill some tetraplegics are able to achieve through intensive training can be quite astounding. In fact, some of them became such expert players that they succeeded in beating paraplegic players with normal function of all the muscles of the upper limbs. Mention may be made here of one of the most excessive forms of readjustment potentialities in the neuromuscular system I have ever seen. This was a young Norwegian with a complete paralysis of all muscles of both upper limbs, including the deltoid and biceps. He learned to play table tennis by holding the bat in his mouth, and he was able both to serve, when the ball was placed on his bat, and to return. During the Games in 1962, to the amazement of all players and spectators, he was able to beat a player of Class 1b.

The Table

The table shall be rectangular in shape, 9 ft long by 5 ft wide. It shall be supported so that its upper surface, termed the 'playing surface', shall lie in a horizontal plane 2 ft 6 in above the floor. It shall be made of any material and shall yield a uniform bounce of not less than $8\frac{3}{4}$ in and not more than $9\frac{3}{4}$ in when a standard ball is dropped from a height of 12 in above its surface. The playing surface shall be dark coloured, preferably dark green and matt, with a white line $\frac{3}{4}$ in broad along each edge. The lines at the 5 ft edges or ends, shall be termed 'end lines', and the lines at the 9 ft edges, or sides, shall be termed 'side lines'.

For doubles, the playing surface shall be divided into halves by a white line $\frac{1}{8}$ in broad, running parallel to the side lines, termed the 'centre line'. The centre line may, for convenience, be permanently marked in full length on the table and this in no way invalidates the table for singles play.

Conditions of Play

All competitors must be in wheelchairs and neither their feet nor their foot-rests may touch the ground during play. Tetraplegics are

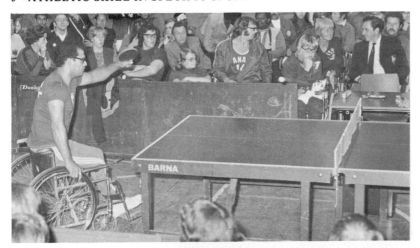

Fig. 65 Table Tennis Singles Final between Israel and U.S.A. at the International Stoke Mandeville Games, 1974.

Fig. 66 Table tennis doubles match. The lady on the right is a complete spinal cord lesion below the 8th cervical segment.

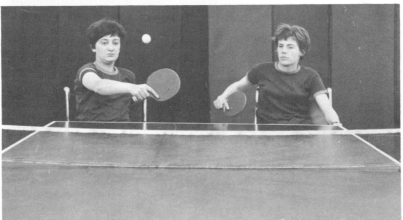

allowed to have the body fixed by a band around the chest or upper abdomen to secure their balance during play. Moreover, they may also secure their equilibrium by slinging the non-playing arm behind the backrest around the vertical bar of the chair.

Clothing

Competitors' clothing shall be coloured but not white or bright coloured. Pullovers, slipovers or cardigans, if worn, should be of the same colour and should not be removed during any one game. Badges may be worn.

General Rules

The rules of table tennis for paraplegics and tetraplegics are in accordance with the official Handbook of the English Table Tennis Association and the International Table Tennis Federation laws with the following additions and amendments:

There will be singles competitions in all classes, with separate events for men and women.

There will be team events in all classes including Class 1 (a combination of Classes 1a and 1b may be necessary).

During play competitors feet and foot rests will not be allowed to touch the floor.

A cushion of any thickness is permitted.

A standard type of chair will be used. If, in the opinion of the referee, a chair has been specially built up for table tennis and would give a definite advantage, the player will be warned by the referee to change the chair and on failing to do this he will be disqualified.

Players are not allowed to sit on any part of the chair except the seat.

Three women and three men will be allowed in each class in the competition.

To make up a team, a competitor may only move down in class.

Mixed unit or country teams are not allowed.

Players are classified in six classes, i e. 1a, 1b, 1c, 2, 3 and 4. Classes 5 and 6 are not included as their small physical deficit enables them to compete in able-bodied competitions.

The server shall first make a good service and thereafter either player on each side shall make a good return.

In order to make up a doubles pair or team a competitor may pair up with a player in his own team and below his own class but not above.

Strict observance of the conventional method of service may be waived when the umpire is notified before play begins that compliance is prevented by physical disability.

A player should not touch the table with his free hand whilst making a stroke but should he do so through loss of balance, the point shall not be counted against him unless he fails to regain his balance prior to making his next stroke (Figs. 65 & 66).

SNOOKER

This game was one of the first to be introduced to paraplegics at Stoke Mandeville during the war and has been practised ever since. Other countries have taken up snooker and it has become one of the regular competitions in the Stoke Mandeville Games, being played also in 1960 in Rome, 1964 in Tokyo, in 1968 in Israel and in 1972 in Heidelberg and it will also be played at the Olympiad in Toronto in 1976.

Although, like precision javelin throwing, it is by no means a dynamic sport, it offers a great variety of movements which promote the paralysed person's mobility and co-ordination and also helps him to develop skilful manoeuvrability in his wheelchair. Above all, it demands the finest precision work, concentration and calculating ability in playing the cue-ball from the

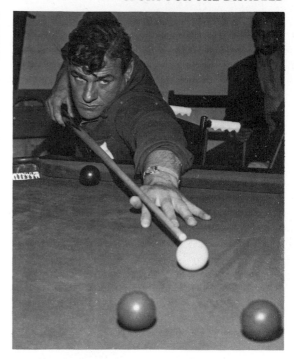

Fig. 67   Snooker match.

position in which it has come to rest to make the right contact with the object balls, whether they are pool balls or reds, with the aim of pocketing them.

Snooker is one of the games where the paraplegic can compete with able-bodied players on equal terms, and such competitions have often taken place (Figs. 67 & 68). Snooker is played on a standard English billiard table, and the general rules, technical terms and laws of the game for paraplegics are the same as in snooker for the able-bodied, authorized by the Billiard Association and Central Council; it is therefore, unnecessary to present the details in this book.

Tetraplegics may make use of a support for the cue which is in the shape of a pyramid with a ring on top through which the tip end of the cue passes. The base of this support is covered with green baize so that it can rest on the table without damage to the cloth.

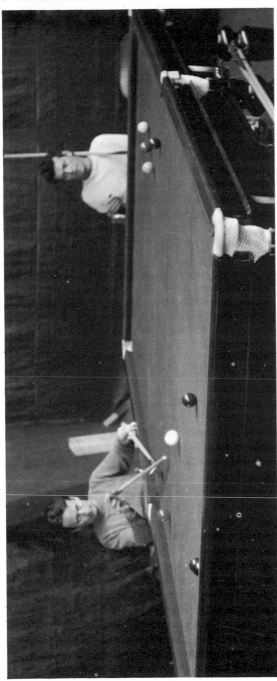

WHEELCHAIR TRACK EVENTS

The track events include wheelchair dash, relay race and slalom and are regular sports events at the I S M G. Skill and standard of performance in mastering ever greater distances with higher speeds has definitely increased throughout the years, commensurate with the provision of better training facilities on large tracks and the use of suitable wheelchairs. At Stoke Mandeville Sports Stadium track events include 40, 60 and 100 metres dashes and 4×40 and 4×60 metres relays but 220 and 400 yards shuttle relays and 880 yards relays have been practised in other countries such as Canada and U.S.A. At the 1976 Toronto, Canada, Olympiad of the Disabled, wheelchair races of 800 and 1500 metres will be included among the competitions. Classifications for track events are the same as for field events.

The Track

The track shall not be less than 7.32 m (24 ft) in width and in all races each competitor shall have a separate lane of at least 1.22 m (4 ft) in width to be marked by white lines, 5 cm (2 in) thick. The track shall be roped off along its whole length. A minimum of six lanes of equal surface should be available. Track surfaces shall be flat, hard and smooth and at least ten yards of unobstructed hard surface shall extend beyond the finish line.

The Wheelchair

The chair should have wheels of not more than 65 cm in diameter and a footstrap of maximum width from 4–8 cm stretched across from the telescopic supports of the footrests or ankle straps on the footrest. A cushion of maximum thickness 10–10.2 cm is permitted. Detachable sides are allowed but must not be removed during the event.

There is still no general agreement regarding the ideal wheelchair for these Games and much

Fig. 68   Snooker match—using cue rest.

has still to be learned. Although there is no doubt that in such races, as in normal track events, the competitor develops his individual style, the type of chair used is nevertheless of great importance. One cannot be too dogmatic about the type of chair used, as one must take into consideration personal preference, but there are certain points which should be uniform to make the competition a fairer one. This applies in particular to the weight of the chair and the size and distribution of the wheels. It would be of course ideal to use special track chairs for racing and slalom but the extra cost would be prohibitive for most competitors. Nevertheless, a specially constructed sports chair has been manufactured in England by Zimmer's, the dimensions of which are as follows:

Height of chair	36 in
" " seat of chair	20 in
Width of seat of chair	17 in
Depth of seat of chair	17 in
Width of chair open	27 in
" " " closed	15 in
Weight of chair	29 lb
Diameter of wheels	24 in

The weight has been cut down by eliminating pushing handles, tipping bars, brakes and side panelling, and by using lightweight foot rests and light materials generally. The sides can be used in the fixed position, swung out by pivoting from the front or detached completely.

Pre-seasonal Training

This comprises exercises in manoeuvrability of the wheelchair, which is particularly important for the slalom, where the competitor has to move his chair in very small spaces. Slow speeds are used at first, which are gradually increased, and starting is also practised. In addition to these specific exercises for racing, gymnastics such as rope work, weighted pulleys or archery should be included to strengthen the shoulder and arm muscles.

Rules for Competition

Wheelchair Races

The Start. A draw for lanes is made at the start of each event, the competitor drawing number one shall take the station on the left facing the winning post, the competitor drawing number 2 the next station and so on.

All races shall be started by the report of a pistol and a start only shall be made to the actual report. The starter should be situated 4 m behind the competitors and shall fire into the air after ascertaining that the time-keepers (one for each competitor) are prepared. The time shall be taken from the flash.

All questions concerning the start shall be with the absolute discretion of the starter, whose decision shall be final.

Competitors must be placed in their respective stations by a marksman. An assembly line marked in a distinctive colour shall be drawn 4 m behind the starting line and parallel to it and across the six lanes. The marksman shall place competitors on the assembly line and signal to the starter when all is ready.

A competitor must not touch the start line or the ground beyond it with his wheels when on his mark.

The start of the race shall be denoted by a line 5 cm wide at right angles to the inner edge of the track and across the 6 lanes. The distance of the race shall be measured from the edge of the starting line further from the finish, to the edge of the finish line nearer to the start, and shall be 50 m or 100 m.

All races shall be started by the actual report of a pistol fired upwards into the air, but not before all competitors are quite still on their marks.

When the starter has received the signal from the marksman he shall give the competitors the following commands:

(a) 'On your marks'

(b) 'Set'. When all competitors are set, i e. motionless on mark, the pistol shall be fired.

If a competitor leaves his mark after the word 'Set' but before the pistol is fired, it shall be considered a false start.

Any competitor making a false start must be warned. If a competitor is responsible for two false starts he shall be disqualified.

If, in the opinion of the starter, the start was not fair, he must recall the competitors with a second shot. If the unfair start was due to one or more competitors 'beating the pistol', it shall be considered a false start and the starter must warn the offender or offenders who shall be disqualified if they continue to offend after one such warning.

Winners of Preliminary Heats. The six fastest times

from the heats shall qualify for the final. A minimum of 10 minutes must be allowed to elapse between the completion of a competitor's heat and the running of the final.

The Race. Any competitor wilfully wheeling near the line with intent to obstruct or touch an opponent to hinder his progress shall be disqualified.

Each competitor must keep in his allotted lane from start to finish. If the referee is satisfied, on the report of a judge or umpire or otherwise that a competitor has deliberately run outside his lane, he shall disqualify him, but if the referee decides that such action was unintentional, he may, at his discretion, disqualify, if he is of the opinion that a material advantage was gained thereby.

If in any race a competitor is disqualified the referee shall have power, in any case where he considers it just and reasonable to do so, to order the race to be re-wheeled, or in the case of a heat, to permit any competitor affected by the act resulting in the disqualification, to compete in a subsequent heat of the race.

No competitor shall be allowed to rejoin a race after leaving the track, either for the purpose of gaining a place or to pace or assist another competitor.

No attendant shall accompany any competitor on the mark or in the race, nor shall any competitor be allowed to receive assistance from anyone during the progress of the race.

The Finish. The finish shall be a line 5 cm wide drawn across the track at right angles to the inner edge and across the six tracks. There shall be 20 m clear at the end of the finishing line. Worsted (white 2 ply Botany) wool shall, if possible, be stretched over this line one metre above the ground and fastened to two white posts placed at each side of the finishing line at least 30 cm from the edge of the track for the express purpose only of assisting the Judges and Referees in placing the competitors.

The competitors shall be placed in the order in which any part of the body (ie. torso, as distinguished from arms, hands or feet) reaches the line across the track or the back of the chair in races in which competitors are wheeling backwards.

A timekeeper will be allocated to each competitor.

Ties. In the event of a tie in any heat which affects the qualification of the competitors to go forward to the final, where practicable, the tying competitors should both qualify.

In the case of a tie for the first place in any final, the referee is empowered to decide whether it is practicable for the competitors so tying to compete again. If he decides it is not, the result shall stand. Ties in other placings shall stand.

Protests. Any protest or objection by a competitor or team against the conduct or placing of another competitor or team shall be made to the referee or judge immediately after the conclusion of that competition. Such a protest or objection shall be made verbally by the individual competitor or by a member of the protesting team. It shall be decided by the referee on the ground and his decision shall be final (Figs. 69 & 70; Table 16).

TABLE 16. Records achieved in Men's (100 m) and Women's (60 m) Wheelchair Dash.

	1970		RECORD	
CLASS	MEN 100 m	WOMEN 60 m	MEN 100 m	WOMEN 60 m
2	29·4 sec	17·8 sec	21·0 sec	16·8 sec
3	24·5 sec	19·1 sec	20·9 sec	15·7 sec
4	26·1 sec	16·9 sec	20·1 sec	15·0 sec
5	27·5 sec	19·7 sec	20·0 sec	15·6 sec

Additional Rules for Relay. Lines shall be drawn across the track to denote the scratch lines (start and finishing lines).

Lines shall also be drawn 10 m before and after the scratch lines to denote the take over zone and no member of a team shall take up a position, or move outside this zone prior to taking over.

The distance of the course shall be 40 m for women and 60 m for men measured from the edge of the starting scratch line furthest from the take-over line to the nearest edge of the take-over line.

The positions of a team at the start of the race shall be drawn and shall be retained at each take over zone.

The take over is only completed and the take over competitor allowed to start when his team mate has entirely penetrated the take over zone and touched his take over on any part of the arm from shoulder to wrist, when the latter has crossed the line indicating the start of the take over area with his leading wheels. The take over may be from a stationary or moving start.

Competitors after completing the course should wheel off the course in their own lane to avoid obstruction to other competitors. If any competitor wilfully impedes a member of another team by running out of position in lane at finish of a stage he is liable to cause the disqualification of his team.

Assistance by pushing off or by any other methods will cause disqualification.

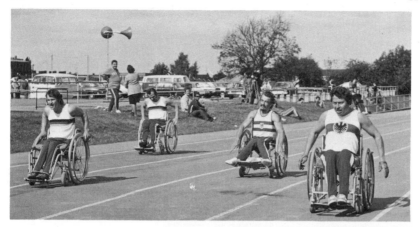

Fig. 69   Men's wheelchair
dash.

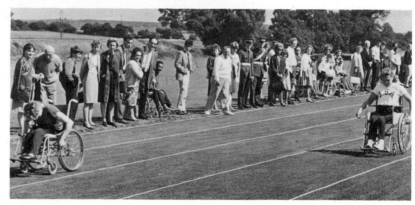

Fig. 70.   Women's wheelchair
dash.

Once a team has competed in the preliminary round of an event, the composition of the team must not be altered for any subsequent round or final except in the case of injury or illness where the referee is satisfied on medical grounds that a competitor is unfit to compete, when he may permit the substitution of another competitor.

It is possible for the order of wheeling to be changed between heats or final.

No competitor may wheel two sections for a team.

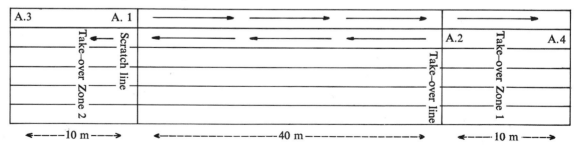

Fig. 71   Diagram of a wheelchair relay course

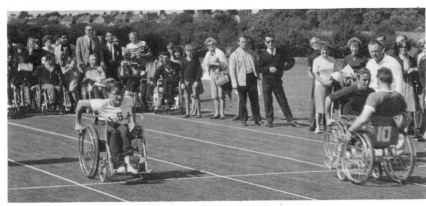

Fig. 72 *Left & below*: A wheelchair relay race in progress.

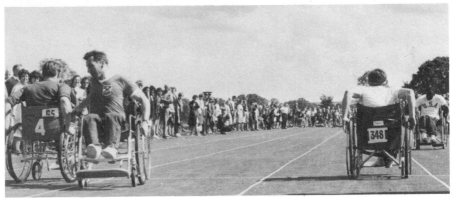

Wheelchair Relay Course

A.1—A.2—A.3—A.4 indicate the members of one team.

A.1 is waiting to start on the scratch line; A.3 is in the take-over Zone 2 behind him in the same lane; A.2 and A.4 are in the take-over Zone 1 at the other end of the course and in the next lane to A.1 and A.3

On the starting signal, A.1. races down the course in his lane and as soon as he has fully penetrated into take-over Zone 1 A.2 can pass over the take over line to dash down in his lane and in turn when he has fully penetrated take-over Zone 2 A.3 can leave the area down his lane and the same with A.4 who completes the course and is timed as he crosses the scratch line (Fig. 72).

Wheelchair Slalom

Classifications are the same as in track events.

While wheelchair dash and relay are speed races which demonstrate the driving power of paraplegics, the slalom is an excellent exercise to improve the wheelchair athlete's co-ordinating power in handling and manoeuvring his chair. It is indeed most illuminating to compare in slalom competitions the great difference in skill and dexterity between the well-trained paraplegic and the others. It is true to say that for the well-trained paraplegic the chair has become the substitute for his legs, and it is fascinating to watch how paralysed athletes succeed in overcoming sometimes very difficult obstacles when negotiating the various gates both forwards and in reverse, with some competitors even tipping up their chairs.

A similar skill in handling a motor car can be observed in the difficult driving tests carried out by disabled drivers in the competitions of the Disabled Drivers' Motor Club.

The wheelchair slalom course comprises a

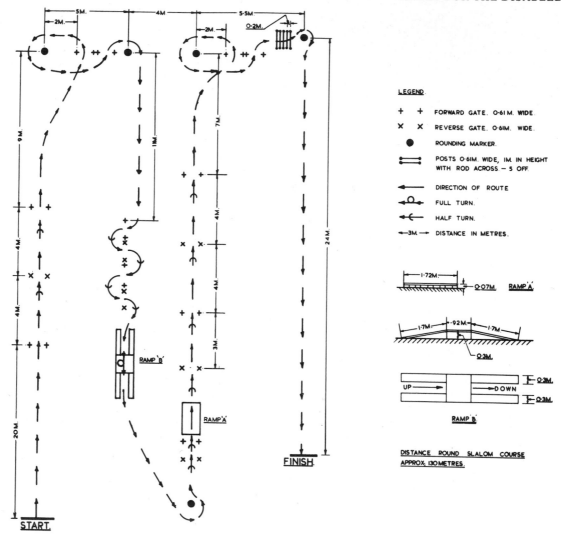

Fig. 73   Diagram of official slalom course for ISMG.

variety of obstacles, consisting of six series of alternate forward and reverse gates. Each series is set out in varying designs which call for the skill of the competitor in manoeuvring first through a forward gate and then immediately through a reverse gate without incurring a time penalty for fouling the gates or passing through in the wrong direction. The width of the gates is 61 cm, with flags marking each side of the gates, different colours being used to distinguish between forward and reverse gates. In one series the gates are set in a straight line (Fig. 73).

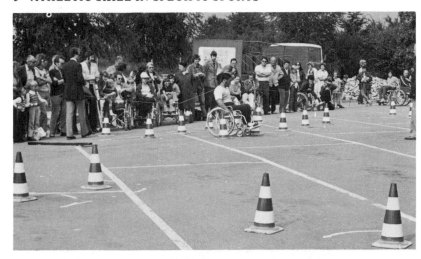

Fig. 74 *Left*: A slalom competition.

Fig. 75 *Below, left*: Reversing through gate in the slalom.

Fig. 76 *Below, right*: Manoeuvring off ramp in the slalom.

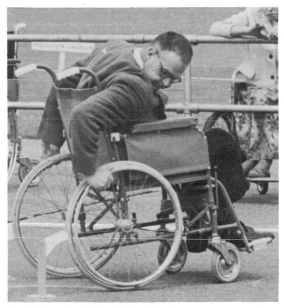

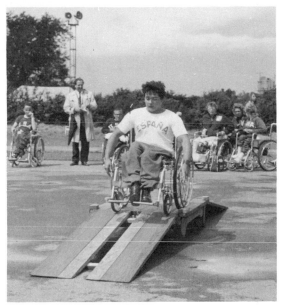

The course also includes three other obstacles, such as raised ramps, etc.

Failure to negotiate the above obstacles correctly results in a time penalty.

The approximate length of the course is between 80 and 90 metres. The time for the distance is noted plus any time-additions for faults.

Where a corner has to be rounded on the course, this is marked by a distinguishing flag.

The layout of the course is altered each year keeping the same basic obstacles (Figs. 74–76).

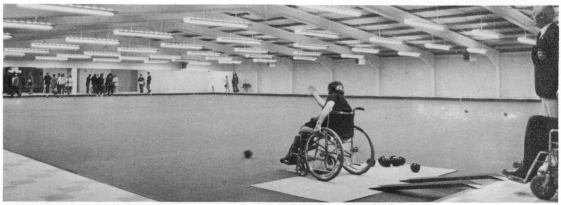

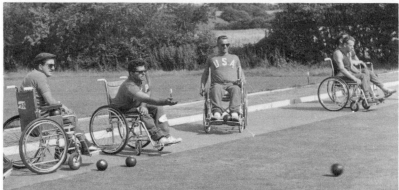

Fig. 77 *Above*: The Lady Guttmann Indoor Bowling Green. Mrs. Gwen Buck, for many years Ladies Champion, at the opening of the Centre. Note the special mat and removable ramp for wheelchair competitors.

Fig. 78 Specially built outdoor bowling green at Stoke Mandeville Sportsground. Note the concrete base for wheelchairs.

Wheelchair Bowling *(Skittles, Flat Green Bowling, Ten Pin Bowling)*

There are no classifications in bowling.

The game of skittles was one of the first forms of clinical sport amongst paraplegic patients at Stoke Mandeville during the Second World War. In those days I also used the game of skittles to bring about the readjustment of co-ordination in hemiplegic soldiers. This sporting activity of paraplegics was later replaced by other sports but once an outdoor bowling green was built, in following years, by the then Paraplegic Sports Endowment Fund, and specifically adapted for wheelchair players by the addition of rectangular concrete layers around the green to avoid damage of the green by the wheelchairs, bowling developed into an integral part of the national and international S M G. In the course of the years paraplegics have become experts in this sport at which the wheelchair athletes can compete on equal terms not only with other physically handicapped, such as the blind or amputees, but also with able-bodied bowlers. Bowling is, indeed, an excellent recreational activity for all age-groups and both sexes and its phenomenal growth has spread to many countries during the last 20 years, not the least by its appeal to the ladies which gives them the opportunity of competing on level terms with the male sex. Bowling has a long history and, like

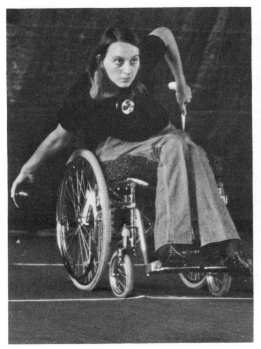
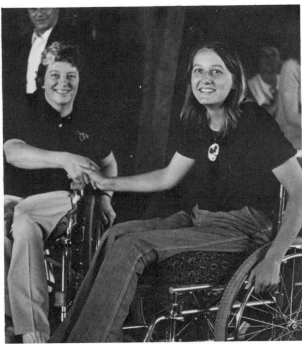

Fig. 79   *Above:* Indoor bowling competition. Mrs Gwen Buck in action, **left**, and being congratulated by a French competitor, *right*, on winning an indoor competition.

Fig. 80   *Below*: Ten-pin bowling match.

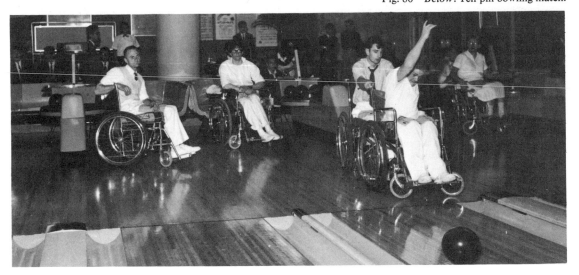

archery, it is among the oldest of English sports. For instance, the Southampton Bowling Club was founded in 1299 and is still active today. Amongst the many references in history to this sport is that famous game played at Plymouth Hoe by Drake, who refused to abandon the game when he received the message that the Spanish Armada was approaching.

The unreliable weather of the English summer, which not infrequently makes bowling competitions for paralysed players difficult, and moreover, the increasing popularity of bowling amongst other disabled and elderly people, were the incentives for the Executive Committee of the British Paraplegic Sports Society to build an indoor bowling green. It was built as a national bowling green mainly by voluntary subscriptions but also with the help of grants given by the Sports Council and the Borough Council of Aylesbury and consists of six rinks. It was named by the Executive Committee of the B P S S "The Lady Guttmann Bowling Green," in memory of Lady Guttmann's great service given to the Stoke Mandeville Sports Stadium and the Games. It was opened in September 1974 by the Mayor of Aylesbury, Councillor Freda Roberts in the presence of Dr. Roger Bannister, former Chairman of the Sports Council, and has been in daily use ever since, including regional and national matches. To enable wheelchair users to participate in indoor bowling two removable ramps and a special mat are available for each rink as shown in Figure 77. Figure 78 shows a match in progress on our outdoor green during the S M G.

The bowls used are of wood or plastic and their sizes and weights must conform to the regulations of the British Indoor Bowling Council, the diameter varying between $4\frac{3}{4}$ to $5\frac{1}{8}$ in. and the maximum weight varying between 3 lb and 3 lb 8 oz.

The technique and rules of bowling for wheelchair users do not differ in any way from those for the able-bodied; they do not therefore need to be described here as they can be learned from the small illustrated book of rules and techniques published by the E.P. Group of Companies, Bradford Road, East Ardsley, Wakefield, Yorkshire, England.

Ten-pin bowling is another form of recreational sport which in many countries, in particular Canada and U.S.A. but also in Great Britain and on the Continent, has been very popular. However, the interest in ten-pin bowling, at least in this country, has recently decreased in favour of the more sophisticated Flat Green Bowling (see Figs. 77–79), the more so as the U.K. Branch of the U.S.A. Brunswick Corporation, which most generously presented the Stoke Mandeville Stadium with a two lane ten-pin bowling alley, has closed down, with the resultant difficulty, in common with other centres, in getting spare parts.

Paraplegics in wheelchairs have taken part in ten-pin bowling contests, and damage to the lanes by the chairs was easily avoided by placing a rubber mat behind the Foul Line. We use three-hole balls of weights varying between 12 and 16 lb and accurate records of the game are made on special score sheets. (Fig. 80).

FENCING

Having had, as a student, personal experience of long-rapier and sabre fencing, including a period as coach in my student fraternity, it occurred to me that wheelchair fencing could be a possible sport for paraplegics and this has proved to be so. Ever since the early fifties wheelchair fencing has been popular amongst paraplegics in various countries and is one of the attractions at the I S M G.

Fencing is a dynamic but elegant sport, which promotes co-ordination and concentration, precision and alertness rather than strength. The three types of fencing practised amongst paraplegics and which are the subject of competition during the Stoke Mandeville Games are foil for men and women, épée and sabre for men only.

Training in wheelchair fencing is as time-consuming for the paraplegic as it is for the able-bodied and requires adaptation to the special needs of the fencer in a sitting position. Any coach can train paraplegics provided he is familiar with the special procedures necessary in wheelchair fencing. It must be remembered that each fencer fights from a chair which is securely fastened to a rigid frame on the floor and therefore at a fixed distance from and a fixed angle to his opponent. Such close quarters require constant concentration and produce a greater strain on the fencer for, unlike his able-bodied counter-part, he cannot retire well out of range for a respite and to relax. This fixed position is similar to that held by German students in long-rapier fencing (Schläger Mensur) where opponents also face each other at close quarters but in a rigid standing position without being allowed even to move their heads, which a judge would considered to be dodging and a foul. The fencing arm is extended straight above the shoulder, and the fencer has to rely mainly on the dexterity of his wrist and hand movements.

Any able-bodied sabreur sitting in a wheelchair and fencing a paraplegic opponent immediately becomes aware of how much more defence normally depends on the feet than the hand. Paraplegics use their trunk, shoulders, arm and hand for propulsion when using their wheelchairs and by training develop great strength in these parts.

The president of a fencing competition may sometimes find it rather difficult to distinguish the beat-attack from the parry-riposte, attack from counter-attack, and to decide whether an attack has been cleared, and he must be familiar with the special rules for wheelchair fencers.

Early in his training the pupil learns to control his weapon in relation to movements of the body, which, as mentioned above, differ considerably from those of able-bodied fencers where movements of the legs play a vital part. At the same time, he learns to appreciate proper timing and to judge distances—important factors for both attack and defence. He is taught a sequence of exercises, starting with very simple offensive and defensive actions, gradually pro-

gressing to a pattern of more complex actions of assault and defence, where he has to learn split-second timing in attack and defence. He has also to develop his own initiative, vigilance and fighting spirit. In due course, when the stability and equilibrium of his trunk and arms have developed the pupil's movements and handling of the sword become less clumsy, and he develops that graceful style so characteristic of fencing, especially the foil. He must also acquire a good knowledge of all the rules, including those of judging. In the past, French and Italian paraplegics, in particular, have excelled themselves in this sport, but in recent years the skill of the British fencers has greatly increased and they are now equal partners to their French and Italian counterparts and hold a very respected position. At the International Paraplegic Games in Rome, 1974, Cyril Thomas won the Gold Medal for Epée Individual and came second in the Sabre Individual against the superb Italian sabreur, Marsen, and the British team won the Sabre team event (Fig. 81). At an international

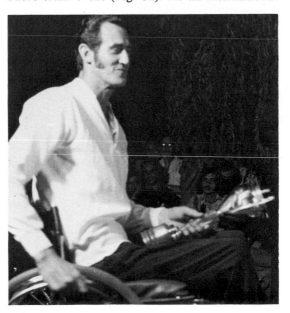

Fig. 81 Cyril Thomas after receiving the team award in Sabre, won by the British team in Rome, 1974.

championship competition organised by the Amateur Fencing Association and held in March 1975 in London, male and female teams of wheelchair fencers gave a demonstration which was well received by both the large audience and the able-bodied competitors.

Rules

The rules for fencing are adapted from the rules of the British Amateur Fencing Association (AFA) based on the rules of the Federation Internationale d'Escrime (FIE) omitting those paragraphs not applicable to paraplegic fencers; paraplegics fencers are, however, advised to study the rule book of the AFA. The amendments made for paraplegic fencers are given hereunder:

General Rules for all three Weapons

Equipment and clothing A fencing frame (Fig. 82) should be provided which conforms to the following specifications:

> 1. It fixes the wheelchair in one position, preferably with a clamp on the outside rear wheels. The whole fencing frame should be clamped firmly to the floor.
> 2. The wheelchairs shall be parallel with each other and at an angle of 15°–20° to the control bar.
> 3. The inside front wheel should be touching the central bar.
> 4. It shall allow for suitable adjustment of the fencing measure to accommodate the three weapons and fencers' arms of varying lengths.
> 5. It should be adjustable to the various widths of wheelchairs.
> 6. For contests with any weapon the inside rear wheels should be covered by round, metal detachable shields.
> 7. If an electric apparatus for signalling hits is used, the metallic piste, wheel guards and the metal parts of the wheelchairs must all be earthed to the apparatus.

Fixed or removable wheelchair armrests are allowed, so long as no part of the armrest on the sword-arm extends higher than the top of the pelvis on that side when the fencer is sitting upright in the centre of the chair. Armrests may be removed. A competitor's feet should not touch the ground during fencing, and his knees must be kept below

FOR FENCERS OF THE SAME HAND

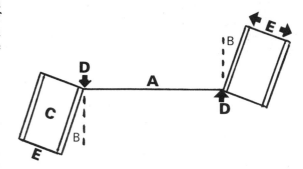

FOR FENCERS OF OPPOSITE HANDS

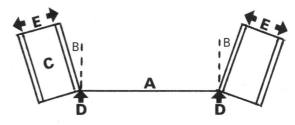

Left hander   Right hander

Fig. 82 Layout and specification of the fencing frame. A. Adjustable central bar; B. Equal angles of between 15° and 20°; C. Whole section adjustable for left-handed fencers; D. Rail allows front wheel to touch the central bar; E. System of rails to allow chairs to be wheeled on, secured and aligned correctly.

the level of his hips. For all weapons the chair must have a back rest of a height of at least 30 cm measured from the seat of the chair without cushions. Cushions must not exceed a total thickness of 10 cm. The legs must be extremely well protected by a plastic apron or extra thickness of cloth. To assist the President in judging the correct fencing measure an arm rest must be used on the opposite side of the wheelchair to the sword-arm. The President will check the heights of the arm rests on the sword-arm side and, with electric foil, the insulation of the wheelchair. With sabre, the President should also check before the competition commences that the 30-cm marks on the wheelchairs are clearly visible.

Positioning for fencing. The fencing frame shall be adjusted before the start of each fight (or later if required by the President) to give the

Fig. 83 Men's Foil competition.

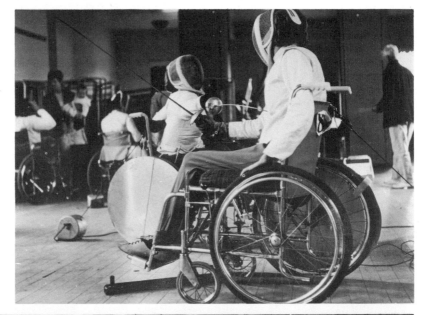

Fig. 84. *Below*: H.R.H. Prince Philip, Duke of Edinburgh, watching a women's fencing competition at the 1958 National Stoke Mandeville Games. In the background is the helicopter which Prince Philip piloted himself.

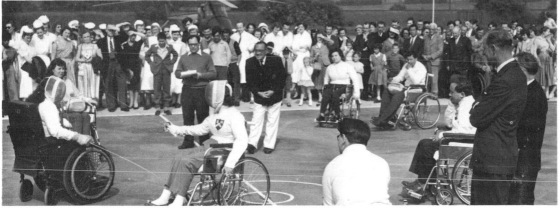

correct measure betwen the competitors. The exact FIE regulations cover the command "Are you ready?" Swords must be stationary until the command "Play".

Foil. The fencers should sit upright in the centre of the width of their chairs with their arms extended towards each other, the points of their foils touching the inside of their opponent's arm. The tip of the blade should be not less than 20 cm from where the seam of the jacket crosses the lower border of the pectoral muscle. A 20-cm measure provided by the Organisers must be used to judge the correct fencing measure.

In the case of fencers of unequal arm-length the fencing measure is that of the fencer with the shorter arm. Where there is a dispute, in particular if the fencer with the longer arm is at a disadvantage, the President may intervene, and his decision is final (Figs. 83 & 84).

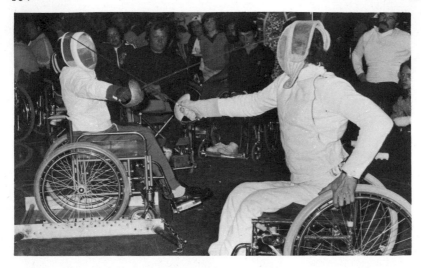

Fig. 85   Épée competition.

Épée and sabre. The same regulation regarding the sitting position also applies to épée and sabre contests, with the exception that with these two weapons one fencer extends his arm and épée or sabre towards his opponent who should have his sword arm bent; in this position the épée should just be able to touch the elbow and in sabre a cut should just be able to be made on the elbow (Fig. 85).

Competitions

It should be noted that this section is not designed as a manual of fencing but is only included in order to help the reader to understand the rules.

1. *Fencing time (Temps d'escrime)* is the time required to perform one simple fencing action.

2. *Offensive actions* are defined as the Attack, the Riposte and the Counter-Riposte.

The attack is the initial offensive action made by extending the arm and continuously threatening the opponent's target.

The riposte is the offensive action made by the fencer who has parried the attack.

The counter-riposte is the offensive action made by the fencer who has parried the riposte.

3. *Defensive actions* are the different parries. The Parry is the defensive action made with the

blade to prevent the attack arriving. Parries are simple, direct, when they are made in the same line as the attack. They are circular (counter-parries) when they are made in a line opposing that of the attack.

4. *Counter-attacks* are offensive actions or offensive/defensive actions made during the offensive action of an opponent.

(a) The stop hit: a counter-attack made on an attack.

(b) The stop hit made with opposition is a counter-attack made by closing the line in which the opponent's attack will be completed.

(c) The stop hit made with a period of fencing time.

5. *Varieties of offensive action.*

(a) The Remise is a simple and immediate offensive action, which follows the original attack, without withdrawing the arm, after the opponent has parried or retreated, when the latter has either quitted contact with the blade without riposting or has made a riposte which is delayed, indirect or composed.

(b) The Redoublement is a new action, either simple or composed, made on an opponent who has parried without riposting or who has merely avoided the first action by retreating or displacing the target.

(c) The Reprise d'attaque is a new attack executed immediately after a return to the on guard position.

(d) Counter time is every action made by the attacker on a stop hit made by his opponent.

Beginning, Stopping and Restarting the Bout

As soon as the command "Play" has been given the competitors may assume the offensive.

The bout stops on the word "Halt". Directly the order "Halt" is given the competitor may not start a new action.

If a competitor stops before the word "Halt", and is hit, the hit is valid. The order "Halt" is also given if the competition is dangerous, confused or contrary to the rules, or if one of the competitors is disarmed, loses his balance or rises from his seat, moves his sitting position, or if the wheelchair becomes unclamped, or if there is any danger to spectators.

Displacement of the target, ducking and half-turns are allowed including raising one slip from the seat.

A fencer may not alter the fencing measure by sliding along and a fencer who does this will, after a warning during the same bout, have a hit scored against him. If during the bout either fencer or the President suspect that the fencing measure has changed, tests must be made and the necessary amendments carried out.

Officials

All bouts of fencing are directed by a President who controls the equipment, including the insulation of the wiring, particularly inside the guard. He supervises judges, ground judges, timekeepers, scorers, etc. and maintains order. He awards the hits and penalises faults. The President fulfils his duty of judging hits, either with the help of four judges or with the assistance of an apparatus for the automatic registering of hits. With the latter, he may be assisted by two ground judges or two judges looking for the use of the unarmed hand. The President and the judges (or the ground judges) constitute the 'Jury'.

Special Rules for the International Stoke Mandeville Games

The FIE rules must be strictly applied during the ISMG in addition to the Special Rules of the present chapter and the modifications listed previously.

Entries must be made on the official ISMG Forms, and must comply with the current ISMG regulations. A country may enter a maximum of three fencers for each individual event and one team for each team event. A team consists of four fencers from whom three are selected for each match. The three fencers must be nominated, at the latest, immediately after conclusion of the individual event of the weapon concerned.

No fencer may compete at more than 2 weapons.

A foilist may fence either as a Novice, if eligible, or in the Senior foil event. A novice may fence for a foil team and, if male, may fence at another weapon.

(*Note*: A novice is one who has never fenced in international competition.)

A country may also nominate, on the entry form, the Team Captain (who may be a competitor but not a member of the Directoire Téchnique or President), one member for the Directoire Téchnique and one or two Presidents at each weapon (who may *not* be competitors).

The Events shall be:

Individual	Team
Men's Foil	Men's Foil
Men's Novice Foil	Women's Foil
Women's Foil	Sabre
Women's Novice Foil	Épée
Sabre	
Épée	

The individual matches must be fought before the team event in the same weapon.

All events should be arranged so that they finish on or before 22.30 hrs.

Professionals may be asked to assist as Presidents, Judges or members of the Directoire Téchnique at the Organising Committee's discretion, until the ISMG get larger.

Organisation

1. The Organising Committee of the Games shall appoint a Director of Fencing (provided by the Host Country) who is responsible for organising all the fencing events and arranging the Juries.

2. The Host Country shall provide all members of Juries except

>> (a) in a team match in which the Host Country is fighting;
>> (b) in an individual Final Pool at Foil and Épée in which the Host Country is represented but all the other participating countries are not;
>> (c) in any Sabre event.

In these cases the Director shall select a neutral President and Jury from the list compiled from the entry forms. Sabre competitors not engaged in a particular sabre pool or match may be used as judges.

Pool/Match sheets, Presidents and Juries should be published in advance.

3. The Organisers shall provide two sets of frames and apparatus for each semi-final and final pool.

A Directoire Téchnique consisting of five members shall be appointed by the Organising Committee of the Games from the list compiled from the entry forms. It must comprise:

>> (a) The Director, who acts as chairman;
>> (b) one other from the Host Country;
>> (c) three others from as many countries as are represented in the fencing events.

In the case of a dispute the Director shall appoint from the Directoire Téchnique a Jurie d'Appel of three persons whose countries are uninvolved. This Jurie d'Appel may decide on interpretations of the official rules, the drawing of pools or matches, or the selection of Juries. All disciplinary action must be referred to the Technical Committee of the Games, whose decision is final.

Countries submitting claims which, in the opinion of the Jurie d'Appel and subsequently of the Technical Committee of the Games, are unnecessary and frivolous, may be excluded from participation in subsequent events in the Games.

Offences and Penalties

Penalties for offences committed by paraplegic fencers are in accordance (with a few modifications applicable to fencers in wheelchairs) with those committed by able-bodied fencers. They are discussed in detail in Articles 623–

657 of the AFA rule-book and should be studied carefully by both paraplegic fencers and officials. The offences are summarised here as follows:

1. *During a contest.* The important offences are: systematically starting before "Play" or after "Halt"; losing balance; rising from the seat; shifting position; moving the legs or coming into contact with the floor; annulment of any hit scored; or altering the fencing measure; at sabre: seeking protection from the back of the chair; and at foil: for protecting or covering the target during the fight with the unarmed arm or hand. Last but not least, any violent action which the President considers dangerous. While hard hits on the paralysed parts of the body may not cause pain, considerable bruising will occur.

2. *Discipline and unsportsmanlike behaviour.* These offences include: failure of competitors' equipment to conform with the regulations; failing to be present when required; any gestures, attitudes or words of a competitor that interfere with the maintenance of good order; refusal to obey immediately the orders of the President, the Jury or other officials, and any other action that offends against the principles of good sportsmanship.

WEIGHT LIFTING

Safety Precautions

As a rule, the sport of weight lifting is suitable for paraplegics with lower lesions of the spinal cord with retained function of the abdominal and lower back muscles.

Before permission is given to a paraplegic to take up weight lifting, he must undergo a thorough medical examination of his lungs and cardiovascular system, which includes measuring the pulse rate and blood pressure, an electrocardiogram, and X-ray of the chest. Anyone who has pathological changes in the lungs and cardiovascular system should be excluded from this sport, as well as anyone suffering from a gastric or duodenal ulcer. An electrocardiogram should also be asked for before the competitions.

Weight lifting is carried out by paraplegics in a lying (supine) position. For safety reasons, an apparatus has been introduced consisting of an adjustable steel rest on either side of the bench fixed in such a way that the cross-bar comes to rest on the outside of the lifter's hands when the bar is lowered. The bar lies 1 inch (2.5 cm) above the chest. To determine the correct height of the bar from the lifter's chest the measuring stick should be placed between the lifter's unexpanded chest, with his arms hanging over the side of the bench, and the lower side of the bar and along the length of the bar which will be on a line with the lifter's nipples. The bar is lowered until the chest, stick and bar touch.

Training

The lifter commences training by just lifting the bar without the weights. Attention must also be given to proper respiration during weight lifting training. Press-on-Bench should always be accompanied by inspiration and lowering the weight by expiration. Once the initial technique is perfected, lightweight presses are started with weights of 11 to 18 kg. The press should be repeated 8 to 10 times. Further progress is made by adding 5 kg to the weight with again 8 repetitions. In due course, heavier weight increases are introduced, using fewer repetitions until the limit of 3 repetitions is reached. If the lifter can only perform 3 repetitions of lifting with his first 5 kg increase, he should remain at that weight and press it from the chest in 4 sets of 3 repetitions or 2 sets of 3 and 2 sets of 2 repetitions. The time to achieve maximum standard naturally depends on the regularity of training, ambition to increase the standard of weight-lifting and proper coaching.

Rules for Competition

Categories
There are six categories of competitors:

1. Light featherweight—up to 50 kg
2. Featherweight—up to 57 kg
3. Lightweight—up to 65 kg
4. Middleweight—up to 75 kg
5. Light heavyweight—up to 85 kg
6. Heavyweight—over 85 kg

At Olympic Games, World Championships, and those contests of a particular Continent or World Zone, six competitors only per country are permitted, spread over the different categories, with a maximum of two lifters per category. *Example*: A country can enter two featherweight, one lightweight, two middleweights and one heavyweight—having no light heavyweight entry; alternatively—two featherweights, two lightweights and two heavyweights—having no middle or light heavyweights.

Weighing-in
Weighing-in of competitors is obligatory one and a quarter hours before the beginning of the competition for a particular category. All the lifters in this category must be present for the weigh-in, which shall be carried out in the presence of the Chief Referee appointed for the category. One delegate of each country with lifters entered may be present. Lifters must strip down to track-suit bottoms; no other clothing or equipment may be worn on the scales (i e. shoes, leg-irons, shirts, etc.). A lifter may weigh in the nude if desired.

Each competitor can be weighed only once. Only those whose body-weight is greater than the maximum or less than the minimum weight in any one class are allowed to return to the scales. They are allowed one hour at the maximum to make the weight. After this time they will be eliminated. A lifter who is too heavy may move into the next higher category if no more than one lifter from his country is entered in this category. All lifters' weights must be recorded exactly.

Technical Rules
The ISMG Committee recognises only one lift (Press-on-Bench) for International and National Competitions and registers World and other international records.

Press-on-Bench. The lifter shall lie supine on an horizontal bench. The lifter's shoulders, buttocks and legs shall remain in contact with the bench throughout the lift; putting the feet on the ground is not permitted. If the lifter is subject to severe spasms of his legs, it is permissible for the legs to be strapped to the bench over the knees. The coach is *not* permitted to speak to the lifter while the *actual lift* is being executed. The use of cushions under any part of the lifter is *not* permitted.

The bar will be placed straight across the lifter's chest, on the stands, and will be horizontal.

The lifter will commence to lift, in his own time, after his name and the weight of the bar has been announced by the MC. At the commencement of the lift, the bar must be in line directly across the chest.

The press movement must be continuous with an even extension of the arms, while the shoulders, buttocks and legs shall remain in contact with the bench throughout the lift. At no time during the lift shall the lifter's upper arms come into contact with the bench. The 'PRESS' is completed when the lifter is motionless with the barbell under control at arm's length. When the Referee observes the lifter in the correct finishing position he will give the signal for the completion of the 'PRESS' which will be the word 'Down', and signal a downward movement with the hand. The lifter will then lower the bar to the stands *under control*. This is the completion of the lift; the lift is not complete until the bar has been replaced on the stands. The Referees will then give their decision and the Chief Referee will confirm the lift by the words "Good lift!" or "No lift!" The Referees' decision is final and cannot be changed.

Reasons for Disqualification
1. Grip too wide.
2. Bar 'stopping' in the press.
3. Uneven extension of the arms.
4. Incomplete extension of the arms.
5. Lifting the shoulders, buttocks or legs off the bench while pressing.
6. Lowering the bar before the referee gives the signal to do so.
7. Dropping the bar heavily, out of control,

onto the stands after the Referee's signal.
8. Any obvious effort to lift must be classified as a lift, and the lift must be classified as 'No lift' if not completed. (An obvious effort is when the bar moves off or along the stands.)
9. Time wasting, which will not be allowed; if a lifter takes too long to lift after his name and weight have been announced (one minute after announcement) he will be 'brought to order' by the Referee, and one more minute only will be granted to 'complete' the lift. Failure to complete the lift in two minutes will bring about the classification of 'No lift', and will be made known by the Referee.

Each lifter is permitted three attempts in a competition. The rising bar method *only* will be used in championships. The weight of the bar will be increased in multiples of 2.5 kg. When the weight of the bar reaches a lifter's particular required weight he will be required to make his attempt. The bar is loaded progressively, the competitor taking the lowest weight lifting first. In no case can the bar be reduced to a lighter weight when a lifter has performed a lift with the weight announced. The lifters, or their coaches, must therefore observe the progressive loading and be ready to make their attempt at the weight they have chosen.

When several lifters declare their wish to make their first attempt with a bar of the same weight, their names shall be drawn by lot. The competitor whose name is drawn first must consequently lift first.

A lifter making his first attempt must precede the lifters taking their second or third attempts with the same weight. Similarly a lifter taking his second attempt must precede any lifter wanting to take his third attempt with the same weight.

In International competitions (except for record attempts made outside the competition) the weight of the bars used must always be a multiple of 2.5 kg. The progression is by 5 kg at a time, a request for 2.5 kg. only indicating the last attempt. The weight shall be announced in kilogrammes and pounds. The weights announced by the speaker must immediately be displayed on an easily visible board.

Should there be an error of loading the bar, or an incorrect announcement, the Chief Referee alone will decide the action to be taken.

The competitor lifting the highest weight to the approval of the referees will be declared the winner. If two competitors lift the same weight, the lighter man is then declared the winner. If both lifters are exactly the same weight at the weigh-in both lifters will then be weighed again and the lighter man declared the winner. If both lifters re-weigh exactly the same then they are declared joint winners and shall both receive a gold award, the silver award being void, and the next highest placed lifter is declared third and is awarded a bronze.

When a lifter announces his commencing weight, he is permitted to change that weight only once, and only to a greater weight. When a lifter is called to the bar to make his selected attempt he must proceed to the area of the competition immediately. If he is not being placed in position on the bench after one minute of being called then he forfeits that attempt. He will not be permitted to attempt the same weight for his next attempt, but must adhere to the law relating to increases of weight between attempts.

If a lifter fails at the weight he selected, he is then permitted to take the same weight again for his next attempt. The minimum increase between first and second attempts shall be 5 kg. If a lifter decides to increase only 2.5 kg after his first attempt, this will constitute his third attempt and he will forfeit his second attempt.

The minimum increase between second and third attempts shall be 2.5 kg. When the lifter is in position to make his effort, then the MC will announce the lifter's name, country, attempt and weight (in kilogrammes and pounds). The lifter MUST make his effort within one minute of the MC's announcement.

Placing of Countries in Final Results

The placing of countries according to their final results achieved is as follows: 7 points are awarded for the first place, 5 for the second, 4 for the third, 3 for the fourth, 2 for the fifth and 1 point for the sixth, but only in World and Continental Championships. If there is a tie, the lighter competitor will be placed before the heavier one to avoid supplementary attempts. For the placing of countries, two lots of 7 points will be awarded for the first two placed, and 4 points for the third place. If there is a tie in the placing, the country having the largest number of first places shall be classified first. If two countries have the same number of first places, that having the most second places shall be placed first, and so on through the third and subsequent places.

World Records

To set up a world record a lifter must perform his lift in front of an official representative of the ISMG Committee and an official of the National association to which he belongs. A registered weight lifting referee (of which there must be three present) is acceptable as a referee to control any record attempted by a paraplegic lifter.

All the Association's rules, as laid down here, must be strictly adhered to, and the controlling referee must be fully conversant with these rules. Two or three favourable decisions count as a 'Good lift'; if only one referee is in favour, this counts as 'No lift'.

As the good faith and competence of the referees of all nations cannot be doubted, the supervision of a world-record attempt can be undertaken by referees of the same nation as the competitor. The conditions to be fulfilled for the registration of a record are as follows:

1. Before making out their report, the three referees must weigh the barbell and the lifter immediately after his performance.
2. The lifter must not leave the platform until he has been weighed.
3. If the record is broken during the course of a public competition, the Chief Referee,

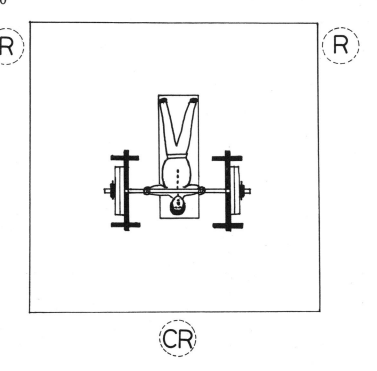

and the Record Registrar, if present, shall have access to the scales.

4. The three referees must draw up a written report, affirming on their honour the validity of the lift, the name of the lifter, his body-weight, the weight of the bar (which must be absolutely precise), the place of the performance, and the date and title of the contest during which the record was broken.

5. This report must be signed by the three referees and the Secretary of the National Federation.

6. A National or International record will only be valid if it exceeds the previous record by at least 500 g (1lb). Fractions of 500 g must be ignored. *Example*: 87.700 kg is registered as 87.500 kg.

7. When a record attempt is made other than at a championship or an organised competition, the lifter and the bar can be weighed before the attempt to avoid the lifter making a wasted effort.

If, in a contest, a lifter narrowly fails to achieve a record (by not more than 5 kg) he may be granted a fourth attempt outside the competition, after that competition is officially closed. In no case will he be granted a further attempt. The report must then be sent to the Secretary of the ISMG Federation, Stoke Mandeville Sports Stadium for the Paralysed and Other Disabled, for ratification by the ISMG Committee.

A record will be valid only for the category at which the lifter actually weighs-in after achieving it. For the purposes of best performances at championships, the face value only of the barbell will be registered, and for that category in which the lifter competed.

Referees
At all National and International meetings there

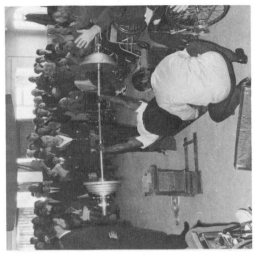

Fig. 88 Press-on-bench by a very spastic paraplegic weight lifter; note the attendant holding his legs.

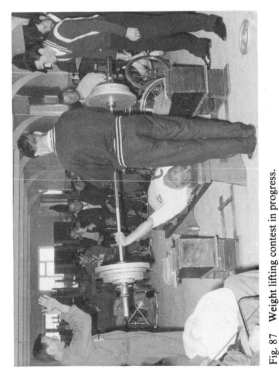

Fig. 87 Weight lifting contest in progress.

should be three referees. One of these, the Chief Referee, controls the contest and gives the signal after the 'Press' to lower the bar to the stands, and makes known the referees' decision. He consults the other two referees and announces the decision based on their opinions and his own by 'Good lift' or 'No lift'. He does not have an over-riding vote.

The Chief Referee shall be seated not more than 4 metres from the centre of the platform and the referees as shown in Figure 86.

Before the contest the referees must ascertain

1. That the platform and equipment are in accordance with the rules.
2. That the scales are accurate.
3. That all competitors weigh in within the limit of their category during the one hour permitted.
4. That the costume of the lifters is correct, as well as the width of their belts (if worn).

During the contest the Referees must ascertain

1. That the weight of the bar agrees with that announced by the speaker.
2. That nobody but the lifter handles the bar during the execution of a lift.

If one of the side referees sees a serious fault during the performance of a lift he may raise his hand to call attention to the fault. If there is agreement from the other side referee or from the Chief Referee, this constitutes a majority opinion and the Chief Referee shall stop the lift and signal to the lifter to lower the bar to the stands. During the contests upon which they are called to adjudicate, the referees must not receive any document concerning the progress of the championship and they must abstain from any commentary.

In international competitions a system of lights arranged horizontally to correspond with the positions of the referees, must be used, which light up only when all three referees press their switches simultaneously and not separate-

In other types of competition small red and

white flags may be substituted for the lights, each referee giving his decision by raising the appropriate flag. In world and other important competitions, referees should be supplied with these flags in case the electrical system should fail.

Referees' decisions are final and there can be no appeal.

Figures 87 & 88 show weight lifting contests at the ISMG and Table 17 lists the records achieved so far by paraplegics.

TABLE 17. Records achieved at Weight Lifting (Bench Press

CATEGORY	1970	RECORD
Light featherweight	115 kg	142·5 kg
Featherweight	141 kg	163 kg
Lightweight	168·5 kg	174·5 kg
Middleweight	170·5 kg	202·5 kg
Light heavyweight	185 kg	197 kg
Heavyweight	215 kg	240 kg

At the 1975 Olympics of the Paralysed at Stoke Mandeville, Brown (USA) established a new world record of 240 kg.

BASKETBALL

Thirty years ago, when we started wheelchair basketball amongst paraplegics, following our successful experiments with wheelchair polo, it would have been quite inconceivable to assume that the time would come when paraplegics could compete in public in this sport not only to their own satisfaction but to the infinite enjoyment of thousands of able-bodied spectators. It is just this sport, which, during the course of the years, has become one of the great attractions of the Stoke Mandeville Games and in sports events amongst the paralysed in many other countries. In the United States, basketball was for many years practically the only organized sport amongst paraplegics, and the skill of the American wheelchair basketball players is particularly advanced, as it is in such other countries as France, Israel, Argentina and Great

Britain. In the ISMG the three best teams were for some years Argentine, Israel and USA, followed by the UK. The UK Team became European Champions (with France second) in 1973 and 1974 (Figs. 89 & 90).

Wheelchair basketball sport is an extremly dynamic game for the paralysed, which brings into play all the adjustment forces in the neuromuscular system and promotes a high degree of integration resulting in complete mastery of the wheelchair. Like soccer, rugby and hockey, it requires not only skill, toughness and endurance but, no less important, team work and team spirit. Above all, it is a sport which demands from every player the highest degree of sensory-motor integration and self-discipline. His behaviour must be beyond reproach to ensure that the game does not deteriorate into an unsportsmanlike scene. The responsibility therefore, of the team leader, as well as of the referees, to enforce the strictest observance of the rules is particularly great. It speaks well for the good sportsmanship prevailing among the paralysed competitors that only once, throughout all the years of the Stoke Mandeville Games, has a team had to be disqualified because of rough play and unsporting behaviour. In our new rule book Articles 76, 77, 78, 79, 81–90 deal specifically with personal conduct and the details of both technical and personal fouls during wheelchair basketball contests, and they should be read carefully by all players, coaches and referees.

As much as the attitude of the players themselves is of great interest from a psychological point of view, so are the reactions of the spectators to this type of sport of these severely physically handicapped. The spectators' reactions are similar to those exhibited at soccer or rugby matches of the able-bodied according to the temperament of the spectators.

Great enthusiasm is also shown in many countries for league competitions and Great Britain, in particular, has a strong league fixture list. The Rules of the SMG apply to these competitions.

Fig. 89 The final basketball
match between Great Britain
and France at Bruges, 1973.

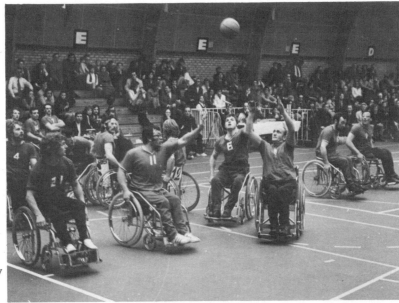

Fig. 90 *Below*, *right*: Terry
Willett, Captain of the British
basketball team, holding the Sir
Ludwig Guttmann trophy given by
the Organisers of the European
Championships at Bruges.

Training

In the training of paraplegics for basketball, five
fundamental activities have to be considered:
wheeling about the court, passing, catching, dribbling and shooting. The training programme,
which involves both individual and team training, is divided into two parts.

Pre-competition Training. This consists of a
series of sessions concerned with diversities of
movement to improve dexterity in manoeuvring
the wheelchair, and may be combined with gymnastics and weight training to improve the
general fitness of the players. These activities include starting, stopping, change of direction,
change of speed of the chair, cutting, pivoting,
revolving, and feinting. Many players are not
very fond of this preliminary training, being
eager to start throwing the ball about. In order
to prevent boredom and loss of interest, it is
wise to include short sessions of ball-throwing
in this stage of training. Training without ball
throwing, however, does help to promote discipline.

Competitive Training. In this period, training
of the individual is directed to dribbling, catch-

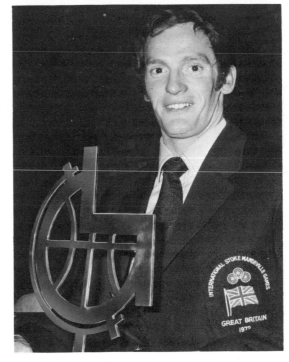

ing, passing, and shooting, and emphasis is given to promoting initiative and skill in individual offensive and defensive actions. This includes guarding the dribbler, stopping the shot and quick action in change of possession of the ball, zone defence and rebounds. Overcoming fatigue and promoting endurance is achieved by gradually increasing the intensity and duration of these exercises. The methods of passing and catching the ball with one or both hands, while the chair is in motion, have to be mastered, and players will develop their own techniques and ingenuity in catching the ball without losing the direction in which they are travelling. Dribbling also demands a great deal of practice in escaping the opponent and advancing with the ball at speed. However, the player must also learn to avoid dribbling if there is a better chance of passing the ball to a fellow player: this develops team spirit. Great skill is required in shooting, especially while the chair is in motion, and various techniques have to be learned, such as set shots in a semi-circle, pivot shots, and throwing the ball backwards into the basket.

Teamwork is, of course, of decisive importance in basketball, and every player must be fully aware of his personal responsibility as a member of the team, both in offence and defence. Only by systematic and continual exercises and practice can co-ordinated team-work develop.

Two methods of defence have to be learned:

(a) man-to-man defence, whereby the ball is of secondary importance, and
(b) zone defence ie. simple zone or combined zone defence. In the latter, training is directed to intercepting and checking an opposing star player by man-to-man defence, while the remainder of the team play zone defence in either square or diamond formation. Team defence is achieved by effective shooting, requiring special skill, both single-handed and two-handed shooting.

A full knowledge of the signals of the referee has to be acquired from the beginning, and last, but by no means least, the referee's decisions must be accepted with self-discipline and courtesy. Even in the heat of the competition, it must never be forgotten that sport is a game and not a war (Figs. 23 & 24).

Rules

Only some of the more important rules can be mentioned here. The rules for wheelchair basketball were amended after the Tokyo Olympics and stood for four years. After the Games in Israel and again after Heidelberg, it was agreed that further amendments were necessary to bring the wheelchair games as close to those of the able-bodied as possible. Details will be found in the recently printed rule book for basketball contests which referees and players taking part in the Stoke Mandeville Games should study carefully and which incorporates the FIBA rules and the amendments necessary for wheelchair play. The most important to be observed in wheelchair basketball are:

the condition of the wheelchair
travelling, dribbling, physical contact, physical advantage
fouls
the numbering of vests and chairs
the change of the six-second rule into a five-second rule.

Contravention of the following rules will result in a chair being banned from the game:

(a) A strap no less than 8 cm in width made of webbing or leather or an elastic strap without metal hooks must be attached firmly and drawn tightly to the telescope bar of the foot-rest platform, so that the bottom of the strap is resting as near to the plates as possible.
(b) Cushions in chairs must not measure more than 10 cm in height, and only one cushion is permissible, sufficiently pliable to allow both ends to meet when folded. Cushions should be the same size as the

seat of the chair. *No* boards or hard materials are allowed in addition to the cushion.

(c) Foot platforms must be exactly 11 cm from the ground at their highest point. Crash bars around the front of the footplates are permitted provided they are exactly 11 cm at their highest point from ground.

(d) All wheelchairs should be fitted with footplates. Blocks on footplates are permitted provided they do not extend over the front of the footplates.

(e) No chairs with additional wheels or rollers will be accepted, which in the opinion of the referee give the player unfair advantage or can be a danger to other players.

(f) The height of seat to be 53 cm.

(g) The referee shall inspect and approve the player's chair.

Points System for Classes taking part

No side shall field a team of more than 11 points. Points are allocated to classes as follows: Class 1–2–3, one point; Class 4, two points; Class 5, three points. This points system gives preference to players with the more severe physical deficits.

Start and Play

The two starting players shall have their chairs in the centre circle, in that half which is nearer to their own basket and with one wheel near the centre line that is between them. An official shall then toss the ball vertically upwards in a plane at right angles to the side lines between the jumpers and to a height greater than either of them can reach and so that the ball will drop between them. Neither jumper shall tap the ball before it reaches its highest point, nor leave their position until the ball has been tapped. Neither of the players taking the jump ball may raise himself from the seat of his chair in order to take the ball.

A player may progress with the ball in any direction within the following limits:

(a) the number of pushes while holding the ball shall not exceed two.

(b) any pivot movements shall be considered part of the dribble and limited to two consecutive pushes without bouncing the ball.

Progress with the ball in excess of these limits is a violation and causes a penalty.

The ball goes into the team's front court when it touches the court beyond the centre line or touches a player of that team who has part of his body or his chair in contact with the court beyond the centre line.

The player who is to put the ball in play from out of bounds shall have his chair with all the wheels out of bounds near the point where the ball left the court. No player must have any part of his body or his chair over the boundary line before the ball has been thrown across the line or put the ball in play after the referee has awarded it to the other team.

Dribbling

A dribble is made when a player, having gained control of the ball:

(a) simultaneously wheels with one hand and bounces with the other;

(b) wheeling and bouncing alternately, placing the ball on the lap (and not between the knees) after either pushing or bouncing. Two bounces followed by two pushes constitutes the legal dribble.

The following are not dribbles: successive tries for goal; fumbles; attempts to gain control of the ball by tapping it from the vicinity of other players striving for it, or by batting it from the control of another player, or by blocking a pass and recovering the ball. An air dribble is illegal.

Violations and Fouls

A violation is an infringment of the rules, the penalty for which is loss of the ball. When an

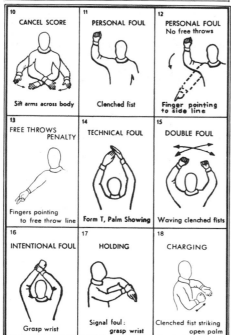

1 TIME IN	2 OFFICIALS TIME-OUT	3 CHARGED TIME OUT
Chop with hand or finger	Open palm	Form T, finger showing
4 SUBSTITUTION	5 JUMP BALL	6 VIOLATION, OUT OF BOUNDS
Crossing forearms	Thumbs up	A. Violations Signal B. Direction of play
7 TRAVELLING	8 ILLEGAL DRIBBLE	9 3 SECONDS RULE INFRACTION
Rotate fists	Patting motion	Fingers sidewards

19 PUSHING	20 ILLEGAL USE OF HANDS	21 TO DESIGNATE OFFENDER
Signal foul: imitate push	Signal foul: strike wrist	Hold up number of player
22 TWO POINTS (One finger—one point)	23 DURING FREE THROWS	24 DURING FREE THROWS
'Flag' from wrist	Signal two throws	Signal one throw

Fig. 91   Hand signals for basketball referees, etc.

10 CANCEL SCORE	11 PERSONAL FOUL	12 PERSONAL FOUL No free throws
Sift arms across body	Clenched fist	Finger pointing to side line
13 FREE THROWS PENALTY	14 TECHNICAL FOUL	15 DOUBLE FOUL
Fingers pointing to free throw line	Form T, Palm Showing	Waving clenched fists
16 INTENTIONAL FOUL	17 HOLDING	18 CHARGING
Grasp wrist	Signal foul: grasp wrist	Clenched fist striking open palm

infringement involves personal contact with an opponent, or unsportsmanlike conduct, the violation becomes a foul which will be inscribed against the offender and a penalty administered.

When a violation is called, the ball becomes dead and is awarded to a nearby opponent for a throw-in from the side-line nearest to the point where the violation occurred. If the ball goes into a basket during the dead-ball period which follows the violation, no point can be scored.

When a player foul is called, involving contact by a player or his chair with his opponent, rising in his chair to gain control of the ball or to gain greater height to handle the ball, taking his feet off the footplate to gain a physical advantage or using a wheelchair which contravenes the rules, the Official shall signal to the Scorer Table the number of the offender and the offending player shall immediately raise his hands and turn to the Scorer Table.

Free Throw. Two free throws are allowed to the offended player after a personal foul.

When a personal foul is called, and a free-throw penalty is awarded, the player upon whom the foul was committed shall be designated by the Official to attempt the free throws.

If the designated player must leave the game because of his injury, his substitute must attempt the free throws. If the player who has been fouled is to leave the game because of a substitution, he shall attempt the free throws before leaving. When there is no substitute available the free throws may be attempted by the Captain or by any player designated by him.

When a technical foul is called, the free throw or throws may be attempted by any player of the opposing team.

The throw for goal shall be made within 5 seconds after the ball has been placed at the disposal of the free-thrower at the free-throw line.

The player who is to attempt the free throw shall take up a position immediately behind the free-throw line with all wheels behind the line, and shall be free to use any system of throwing the ball, but he shall not touch the free-throw line or the court beyond it until the ball touches the ring, or the basket, or the backboard.

When a player is attempting a free throw, the other players shall be entitled to take the following positions:

(a) two players from the opposing team, the two places nearest the basket;
(b) all other players may take any other position, provided that:
(i) they neither disturb nor are in the way of the free thrower and any of the Officials;
(ii) they do not move from their positions before the ball has touched the ring;
(iii) they do not occupy the places along the free-throw lane next to the end line.

Officials' Signals
The hand signals illustrated in Figure 91 should be learned thoroughly by coaches, referees,

scorers, timekeepers and, above all, by the players themselves.

PENTATHLON

This competition has been included in the Stoke Mandeville Games for many years and is still

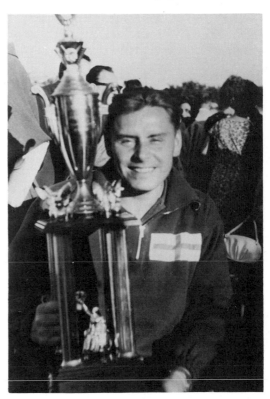

Fig. 92 Dick Thompson, MBE, ten times winner of the Pentathlon trophy in National and International competitions.

very popular (for the classes taking part, see the section on the classification of physical handicap in Chapter 4). Three male and three female competitors shall be allowed for each unit or country and there are separate competitions for men and women in all classes (Fig. 92).

All events must be completed in two days and at the time laid down for each event. If one event has not been competed in, all previous events will be declared void and any remaining events cancelled.

The rules will be the same as those set up for any particular event.

Sports Events for Pentathlon

1. *Archery*

    48 arrows at 50 m on 122 cm face using 5-zone scoring.

2. *Javelin* (women's Olympic model) *or Club*

    (a) Classes 1c, 2, 3, 4 & 5 will be allowed to throw three javelins, the best of three to count.

    (b) Classes 1a & 1b will be allowed to throw three clubs, the best of three to count.

3. *Shot Put* (Classes 1a, 1b & 1c—2 kg shot; other classes, women—3 kg shot, men—4 kg shot.) All classes will be allowed three attempts, the best of which will count.

4. *Wheelchair Dash* Women, all Classes—60 m
    Men, Classes 1a, 1b & 1c—60 m
    Men, Classes 2 & 5—100 m.

5. *Swimming* Free Style Classes 1 & 2—25 m
    Classes 3 & 4—50 m
    Classes 5 & 6—100 m

6

Sports for Amputees

General Considerations

Many of the sporting activities of amputees, especially leg amputees, are carried out with the use of a prosthesis. It is, therefore, absolutely imperative to develop skill in the use of the prosthesis, as it is in the use of a wheelchair for paraplegics, and certain remedial exercises, including sporting activities, can be utilised advantageously in the training of prosthesis users. One of the most deplorable shortcomings in the rehabilitation of amputees, both before and after the second World War, was the failure by hospitals to provide sufficient training for the amputee in the proper use of his prosthesis, and this applied both to arm and leg amputees; it was taken too much for granted that by trial and error the amputee would eventually learn to use his prosthesis satisfactorily. The result of this mistake was frequent discontent amongst amputee ex-servicemen in this and other countries, and their organisations—in Great Britain in particular, BLESMA—took the initiative to organize re-training courses in training centres. However, the situation has now improved; research for the most suitable prosthesis is still continuing and with it has come an awareness of the need for better facilities for training in the use of the prosthesis. It is now generally realised that, just as a paraplegic must not only be provided with the most suitable type of wheelchair and calipers, but must also be well trained in the use of these aids to enable him to lead an active and useful life, the same applies to the amputee with his prosthesis.

Before the amputee is discharged from hospital, he is referred to a limb-fitting centre for measurement for a prosthesis. There are several such centres in UK, the most well-known being that at Queen Mary's Hospital, Roehampton, London. A period of some weeks and even months may elapse before the prosthesis is finished, fitted and adjusted. During this period, a programme of systematic adjustment exercises to the amputation has to be organised by the hospital or training centre as a precondition to the successful use of the prosthesis. It is important to bring the amputee's relatives into the programme, as their help will be needed. They must be instructed in the technique of bandaging and exercises as well as in the hygiene and care of the stump, although the amputee himself whilst in hospital is taught the details of management of his stump.

The amputee's artificial limb must fit in harmony with his body, as any discomfort inevitably leads to disturbance of posture and gait resulting in increased effort, early fatigue and deformities. It is obvious that the higher the arm or leg amputation the more serious becomes the problem of adjustment.

A prosthesis is subject to sudden strains and stresses during exercises and sport, and to wear and tear. It is therefore desirable that the amputee should be trained in the anatomy and construction of his limb and instructed in its servicing and in minor repairs, which will help to prevent major breakdowns and minimise repair and servicing by the limb-maker.

Classification

Amputees were originally divided by I S O D into 27 classes according to their individual physical deficits. However, this detailed classification not only made it impossible in practice to organise competitions for amputees on such a large scale, but the number of competitors entering in each category was insufficient to provide satisfactory competition. Because, from the medical point of view, it is possible to combine some of the categories without disadvantage to the competitors, the Praesidium of ISOD has, therefore, after full discussion, reduced the original 27 categories to 12, which will be subject to review after the 1976 Olympiad in Toronto.

The 12 categories are as follows. The former Classes A, A1, B, B1, G—G4, H—H3, I—I2, J—J1 and K have been abandoned as individual classes and combined with others into a new series of Classes A—F, as shown in Table 18.

TABLE 18. Amputee Disability Classification

Class A	Single BK: Single BK+Forepart foot: Pirogoff on one side: Forepart foot+ *Pirogoff.*
Class A1	*Double BK*+Pirogoff both sides: Single BK+Pirogoff.
Class B	Single AK: Single AK+Forepart foot: Single AK+Pirogoff.
Class B1	Double AK: Single AK+BK.
Class C	Single BE: Single BE+Forepart foot.
Class C1	Double BE: BE+AE.
Class D	Single AE: Single AE+Forepart foot.
Class D1	Double AE.
Class E	BK+BE: BE+Pirogoff.
Class E1	BK+AE: Single AE+Pirogoff.
Class F	Single AK+Single BE.
Class F1	Single AK+AE.

Abbreviations BK—below knee amputation
BE—below elbow amputation
AK—above knee amputation
AE—above elbow amputation

TRAINING AND COMPETITIONS FOR ARM–AMPUTEES

Preliminary Training

Amputation of one arm, especially above the elbow, invariably results in deformities of the shoulder and spine, especially if no prosthesis is worn. The shoulder on the side of amputation is elevated as a result of unrestrained action of the levator scapulae and trapezius muscles, and if not counteracted by appropriate exercises from the start, this unrestrained action and the counterweight of the normal arm causes increasing elevation of the shoulder, resulting in more or less profound sciolisis of the spine. Wearing an arm prosthesis is in itself a useful measure in preventing or at least diminishing the deformities of the shoulder and the trunk. However, stump gymnastics with and without prosthesis are invaluable in preventing atrophy of the stump muscles by greatly improving the circulation in the stump and increasing the strength and volume of its remaining muscles. The purpose of resistance exercises, such as with pulleys, weights, metal expanders and the carrying of a sandbag of increasing weight with the stump elevated forwards and sideways, is to strengthen those muscles which counteract the overaction of the elevators of the shoulder, and to strengthen the depressor muscles of the shoulder, especially the pectorals, latissimus dorsi and serratus anterior. Ball games with the stump and, in particular, swimming are invaluable in developing good mobility of the stump. Throwing a medicine ball from different directions is useful in this respect especially for double amputees. Below elbow amputees can, with advantage, carry out swinging exercises on parallel bars, and there is no reason why upper arm amputees should not perform certain gymnastics with special gadgets fixed to their prostheses to ensure a safe grip on the bar or rings, especially in the case of patients who prior to their amputation were skilled gymnasts.

Athletic skill in Specific Sports

Swimming

This sport is enjoyed by many arm amputees, including high double-arm amputees. Those who were experienced swimmers before amputation can adjust themselves very quickly to their new

condition. They will naturally adopt a favourite
stroke by specialized training, in accordance
with their handicap, once they take up swimming as competitive sport.

The main strokes which the amputee will be
likely to use are the back stroke, breast stroke
and crawl. In all strokes, the legs will perform
the main work in propelling the body through
the water.

Back stroke. Arm amputees usually start with
the back stroke, letting themselves glide backwards into the lying position in the water from a
standing or half-kneeling position, by pushing
the legs from the ground and keeping the trunk
in extension.

One-armed amputees who commence swimming by throwing both arms backwards will
first overact with the normal arm, and this may
initially result in deviation of the body towards
the normal side. However, this overaction can
be compensated for by increasing the work of
the leg on the side of the arm amputation and
this will enable the amputee to swim in a
straight course. Only if the leg on that side is
also incapacitated by amputation, contractures
in hip and knee joints, or paralysis, will that
compensatory function be absent or greatly
diminished, and may result in the swimmer
taking a diagonal line or a circle. However, evidence has already been presented in the chapter
on the swimming training of paraplegics of how
even a high one-armed amputee associated with
a complete high thoracic paraplegia can be
trained to adjust himself to enjoy swimming an
almost straight course. This was achieved by ex-
tensive training of the stump itself, and with the
aid of a frog-arm to counteract the overaction of
the normal arm. Moreover, the normal arm had
also to adjust itself to the new condition by not
pulling sideways from the forward extended
position but obliquely downwards under the
body. However short the stump may be, it must
never be allowed to remain inactive during swimming. Therefore, even double-arm amputees
where the amputation involves the shoulder
joints can safely use the back stroke once they

are trained. The trainer's position in this case
will at first be behind the amputee, and he must
support the back of the amputee's head as in the
early training of tetraplegics.

Breast stroke will hardly present any serious
difficulties in double-forearm amputees, especially those where only the lower third is
affected. The arm technique in using the stumps
will be similar to that used in the butterfly
stroke. Double-arm amputees above the elbow
will, however, have greater difficulty in keeping
the head above water and must compensate for
the loss of the function of the arms by increased
extension of the trunk. Therefore, well-trained
double-arm amputees may do the same as
demonstrated previously with the well-trained
tetraplegic below C6–7, namely, to swim
several strokes under water and then raise the
head out of the water to breathe.

In the crawl, where the main work is done by
the arms, distal forearm amputees will have
little difficulty, especially if the legs provide a
strong propelling force. However, higher double-
arm amputees will encounter difficulties, with
this stroke, even in the back crawl. Whether the
Krukenberg stump offers advantages in swimming over other stump forms, as stated by
Lorenzen, needs further investigation.

The introduction of the frog-arm has been a
great help in facilitating swimming by arm amputees, especially those with high arm amputation. As shown in our own arm amputees associated with high thoracic paraplegia and tetraplegia, it has proved invaluable in improving the
function of the stump and enabling those with
even the most excessive handicap to swim an
almost straight course. Frog-arms have been particularly useful for the back stroke in these
severely physically handicapped patients.

Swimming Contests (without prosthesis)
The following contests are practised:
  1. Individual entries: 100 m with dive start
  for breast stroke, crawl, back crawl,
  butterfly and free style.
  2. Multi-style individual: 50 m breast

stroke, back crawl, crawl, butterfly.

3. Relay Team (4 persons): 50 m breast stroke, crawl and butterfly, all 4 times.

4. Multi-Style Relay: 50 m breast stroke, crawl, back crawl and butterfly (all once only).

Competitors should not be required to swim more than two events. One hour should be allowed between events.

Diving
This is certainly practised by many arm amputees, especially those who previously engaged in

this sport. There is no doubt that most one-arm and double-arm amputees can achieve great skill in diving, even from the high springboard, and I have witnessed forward, backward and somersault diving of these physically handicapped at a sports festival organized some years ago in Heligoland by the German Sport Association for the Handicapped (D V S), which I attended as a representative of the World Veterans Federation.

Whilst paying tribute to the courage, endurance and skill of these athletes, the dangers of diving cannot be stressed too much, and the amputee must realise that diving can be very adventurous. Strict precautions must therefore be taken by all concerned with diving sports to prevent accidents such as hitting the head against the floor of the swimming pool or against the bed of a river or lake after diving from a rock or boat, which can easily lead to fracture dislocation of the cervical spine and result in tetraplegia. It is absolutely imperative that, during diving training and competitions for amputees, at least one if not two attendants be constantly in the water to supervise the exercise, and care should be taken that no other swimmers are in the neighbourhood of the diver. The warning which I have given in all my lectures to the able-bodied not to indulge in diving in rivers and lakes of unknown depth and in rough seas with

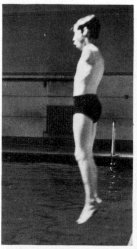
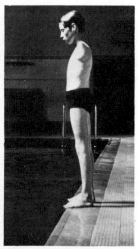

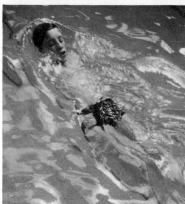
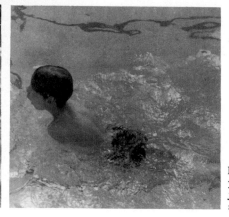

Fig. 93 Congenitally armless youngster demonstrating the jump start and swimming back stroke and breast stroke.

high waves is also applicable to amputees to prevent further increase of their existing disability. As mentioned before, amongst the cases of traumatic tetraplegia, diving accidents amongst able-bodied swimmers rank even higher than industrial accidents and are second only to road accidents. Therefore, instructors must be absolutely aware of their particular responsibility when supervising diving training and competitions for amputees. So far as I am aware, however, no serious accidents have been reported in this particular sport for amputees.

Starting and Turning
Special consideration must be given to starting and turning. In the breast stroke, crawl or free-style, arm amputees start by jumping from a standing or crouched position from the edge of the pool or starting block, and it is important that they should learn to keep the normal arm in such a position as to avoid torsion and rotation of the body when hitting the water. Double-arm amputees have less tendency to rotate. Starting for back stroke and back crawl is best done in the water. The younger the armless swimmer the sooner will he learn to dive-start into the water for either breast or back stroke. Fig. 93 shows a young boy born armless who became an excellent swimmer, diving into the water and using both breast and back strokes. The Amputee Section of BSAD includes young amputees as a special group, which was founded by Len Sofley, an amputee from the second World War and a member of BLESMA. Special training is necessary for double-arm amputees, especially those whose amputations involve the shoulder joints and for whom the propelling force depends entirely on their legs, in learning to avoid collisions with other swimmers and the wall of the swimming pool. It takes some time for double-arm amputees to learn to use the compensatory neuro-muscular mechanisms of the trunk, pelvis and legs to achieve appropriate and timely turning movements of the trunk coordinated by proper function of the legs and thus avoid collisions. I

know of at least one double-arm amputee who, not having acquired the necessary skill in proper turning movements, hit his head against the wall of the swimming pool. On the other hand, a highly skilled double-arm amputee swimmer can train himself to avoid collision by calculated above and underwater turning away from the obstacle, just as a fish would do. To avoid accidents during back stroke swimming by double arm amputees, Lorenzen suggested reducing the usual distance of 50 metres to 30–40 metres by fixing a line across the pool under which the competitor could swim and turn without touching the edge of the pool. We did not find this precautionary measure necessary in our 25-metre swimming pool and turning for

TABLE 19. Competitions open to Bi-lateral Forearm Amputees

Individual entries	1. 50 m breast stroke and free-style wtih dive start.
	2. 50 m back stroke with start in water.
	3. 100 m multi-style: 25 m back stroke / 50 m breast stroke / 25 m free style
Team entries:	50 m breast stroke / 50 m freestyle } 4 times
Multi-style	25 m back stroke / 50 m breast stroke / 25 m free style } once only

50-metre contests was carried out satisfactorily by high double amputees. Thalidomide children without both upper limbs who regularly take part in the national competitions of BSAD have become such excellent swimmers by compensatory function of their legs that they can compete successfully with much older competitors having double upper limb amputations.

One-arm amputees have, of course, little difficulty, if any, in turning properly during breast stroke, back stroke and crawl competitions.

Field Events

Most of the field events are very suitable sports for one-arm amputees, in which they can achieve considerable skill. Although these sports are carried out with the normal arm, the whole body including the stump is trained in the development of a new scheme of co-ordination. One-arm amputees who seriously take up field events, such as distance javelin throwing, shot put, throwing the club, and discus, as a competitive sport have to develop specific muscular strength to achieve greater force and produce greater release velocity. They will therefore have to include in their training for these specific sports progressive resistance weight-training, using dumb bells, punch-balls, and balls of known weight. This type of weight training has the advantage that, in contrast to press-ups, wood-chopping, medicine ball etc., it allows the athlete to measure more accurately his improvement in strength, which, of course, also has a beneficial psychological effect. Like able-bodied sportsmen, arm amputees will also have to strengthen their leg, hip and trunk muscles.

Javelin

Evaluation and measuring. A men's javelin is 230 cm long and weighs 800 g.; that for women is 220 cm long and weighs 600 g.

a. A curved throwing-line with an arc 4 m long and inner radius of 8 m, comprises the boundary which the thrower must not cross. It supports the 7 cm-wide starting-line which must be sunk into the ground and marked with white paint.

b. The course, so far as its dimensions can be expressed by the regulations, must be 35 m long and 4 m wide and the maximum limits must be marked up to the starting point. The last 8 m of the approach must be specially strengthened.

c. An 80–90 m segment at an angle of 29° comprises the field of action. Its lateral extent must be marked out with chalk lines which, if produced, would meet at the centre of the circle (Fig. 94).

d. Whether or not the javelin 'sticks' or remains lying horizontally (provided always that the point is directed forward) the zero point of the tape-measure must be placed against the rearmost position. The distance to the centre of the circle, as measured as far as the inner edge of the starting line, gives the result of the throw.

Both distance and precision javelin throwing are practised. Unlike the chair-bound sportsman, the one-armed amputee has to acquire the technique of the able-bodied in distance javelin

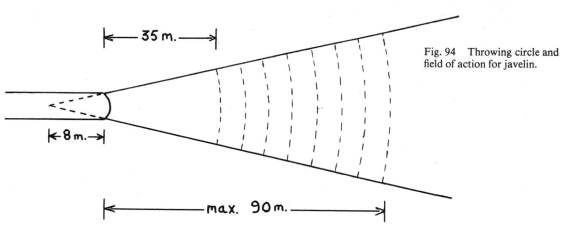

Fig. 94   Throwing circle and field of action for javelin.

throwing and has to learn to adjust his posture accordingly. From the beginning, he must take care not to allow the tip of the javelin to deviate from the straight direction of throw and to release the javelin when the throwing end has reached the highest point above the shoulder. He will also have to develop a new scheme of counter-balance on the side of the amputation to acquire correct equilibrium during the throw.

Training. Training in javelin throwing starts from the standing position to give the athlete an idea of the position from which he should throw, followed by throwing during walking, then throwing with a shortened run, until finally, walking, running and throwing are co-ordinated. The final stage should be attained as soon as possible and the progressions should all be completed efforts (Fig. 95).

Precision javelin, which was first introduced in Germany for one-armed amputees, has also become popular in wheelchair sport. Amputees throw the javelin from a distance of 12 metres for Classes E–F from a standing position, which demands great concentration, co-ordination and accuracy. The circular target is the same as for precision javelin for paraplegics. The distance from the centre of the target to the throwing line is 15 metres for men and 12 metres for women.

Throwing the Club

This is one of the sports in which the one-arm amputee can achieve great skill and compete with able-bodied athletes. The design and weight of the club is the same as shown in Fig. 58 for chairbound athletes. Care should be taken from the start to avoid overhead throws. Throwing the club is practised either from a standing position or with a run-up. The approach run, throwing field and method of measurement are the same as those for throwing the javelin.

Shot Put

The weight of the shot for men is 5.5 kg and for women 4 kg. Fig. 96 is a diagram of the throwing arrangements for the shot put.

Starting Circle.

a. The starting circle (E) must have an interior diameter of 2.135 m (A) and must be outlined by means of a circular mark 76 mm high and 6 mm thick. This must be either an iron or steel ring, the inner surface of which must be faced with concrete and must be 2 cm below ground level. The ring must be marked in white paint.

b. The dimensions of the starting beam, which must be firmly fixed to the ground to outline the front portion of the circle, must be: 1.22 m long, 10.02 cm high and 11.04 cm wide. Metal angles must be used to fix it, or threaded bolts or sleeves sunk into the concrete. The circle itself is painted white.

c. *Evaluation and measuring methods:* The put is disallowed if the competitor, after beginning it, touches the ground outside the circle with any part of his body,

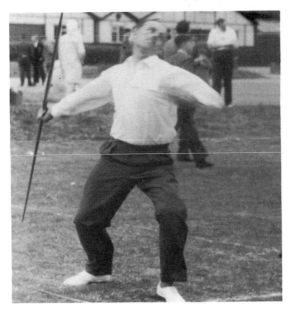

Fig. 95 A one-armed amputee competes at javelin throwing.

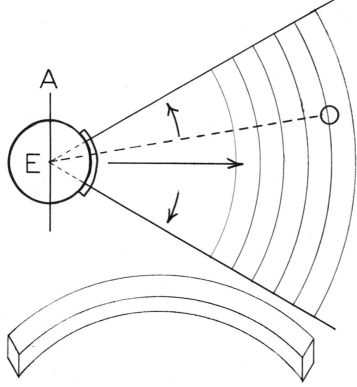

Fig. 96   Shot put. *Upper*: Throwing arc and projection *Lower*: Stop board.

or if he steps on the edge-line. He must leave the circle backwards from a secure standing position behind the centre-line, as marked. (The rear half of the circle must be clearly marked with chalk.) The shot must fall within a 65° sector, measured from the centre of the circle, the limits of which must be marked on the ground extending outwards from the edge of the circle as shown in Figure 96. The length of the put is measured between the point on the shot nearest to the starting circle and the edge of the circle, by extending the measuring tape from the shot towards the centre of the circle and reading the distance at the point where it crosses the inner edge of the starting line.

Training. Those one-arm amputees who have

had training in this sport prior to amputation will adjust themselves to their new condition in a short time and will regain their technique. Beginners start their training in the shot-put with certain gymnastics which include supination and pronation movements of the hand, swinging movements in various directions, including circular arm movements of the arm holding the shot, throwing the shot upwards and catching it, etc. This is followed by training in the actual throwing technique which is carried out from a radius of 3 metres and includes correct holding of the shot, standing put (with right knee bent and body leaning to the right, with shoulders turned to face back of circle—hardly any weight on left foot) stretching right leg vigorously and driving knee to front, stretching right side of trunk, throwing right shoulder high and well forward, finishing with easy action

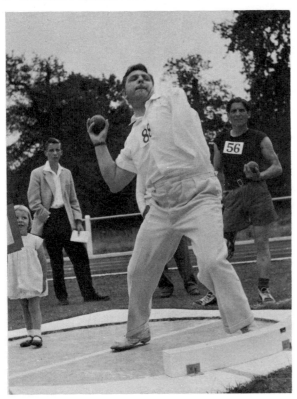

Fig. 97 One-armed amputee putting the shot from a standing position.

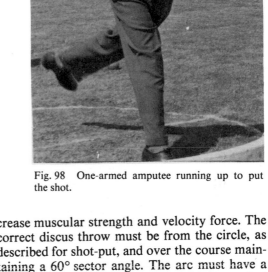

Fig. 98 One-armed amputee running up to put the shot.

of throwing arm, straightforward swinging of the left leg in the right-hand throw and the appropriate associated movements of the trunk. The opposite applies to a competitor throwing with the left arm. Care should be taken that the action of the put is not a straight one (Figs. 97 & 98).

Discus

The weight of the discus is 1.5 kg for men and 1 kg for women. This is also a suitable sport for one-arm amputees, which, however, requires systematic training to maintain the balance during the powerful swinging movements of the arm, trunk and head. As in shot-put and club throwing, weight training is also essential to in-crease muscular strength and velocity force. The correct discus throw must be from the circle, as described for shot-put, and over the course maintaining a 60° sector angle. The arc must have a diameter of 2.50 m. The surface must be marked by means of a circle 7.6 cm high by 0.6 cm thick, looking outwards. The ground within the circle must be 2 cm below that of the exterior (Figs. 99 & 100, p. 128)

Tennis—Table Tennis—Squash Racquets

There is no reason why a one-arm amputee should not enjoy tennis as a sport and, with proper training, achieve considerable skill. In fact, there are amputees who have successfully

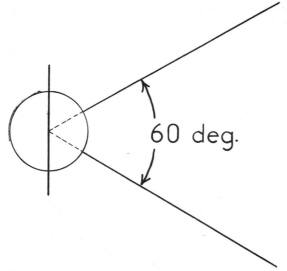

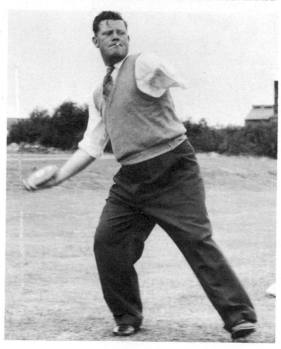

Fig. 99   *Above*: Discus throwing circle and projection.

Fig. 100   *Above, right*: One-armed amputee competing in a discus competition.

Fig. 101   *Below*: One-armed amputee competing at table tennis.

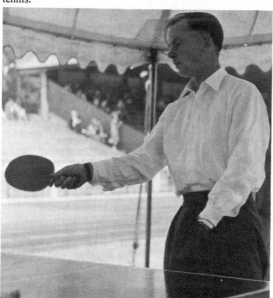

competed with able-bodied tennis players. In this connection, the Austrian tennis player Redl, who lost his tennis arm and trained afterwards with the other arm, again achieved great skill and became champion several times, being amongst the first 16 at the international tennis championships at Wembley in the fifties. However, it must be admitted that the number of amputees who have taken up this sport is very small.

Squash Racquets is a sport which is not frequently indulged in by one-arm amputees, but it is certainly one to improve all-round fitness.

In contrast, table tennis is one of the most popular games amongst amputees. Although the majority of arm amputees, including forearm amputees, use the normal arm in this sport as shown in Fig. 101, there are some who have acquired considerable skill in playing with the stump either with or without a prosthesis. In this connection, the Krukenberg arm seems to be particularly suitable. Below elbow amputees

without the Krukenberg arm can, like tetraplegics with paralysis of their finger muscles,
play by having the bat fixed to their stump.
Table tennis has proved invaluable in promoting
strength and dexterity of the stump. One-arm
amputees who play with their normal arm have,
of course, little difficulty in competing against
able-bodied players.

Golf

This sport is much practised amongst amputees,
particularly in the English speaking countries.
Mention has already been made (page 17) of the
British Society of One-Armed Golfers and the
National Amputee Golf Association of
America, which includes both arm and leg
amputees. One member of the British Society is
a paraplegic who started to play one-handed at
the age of 60, and being a very keen player was
appointed Captain of his local Club. The
players play with the normal arm and the rules
of the Society formally state: "In all
competitions organized by the Society of One-
Armed Golfers, all persons taking part must play
every stroke with the one arm, any aid or
artificial appliance or stump or part of the arm
being barred".

In his article *Playing Golf with One Arm*
R.D. Marshall (1961) distinguishes four different
ways of playing golf with the normal arm.

Right Arm
   A. Forehanded (with right-handed club)
   B. Backhanded (with left-handed club)

Left Arm
   A. Forehanded (with left-handed club)
   B. Backhanded (with right-handed club)

Most right-handed players use a forehand
stroke, while most left-handed players use a
backhand stroke. The general opinion is that the
backhanded player can hit a longer ball but that
the forehanded player is more accurate around
and on the green. According to Marshall, almost
all British One-Arm Golf Champions were
forehanded players but, in recent years, the

backhanded players have become predominant.
With constant training, a few players have succeeded in playing the long shots backhanded
and the shorter game forehanded.

The techniques of playing are principally
identical to those of normal golf, and the training and rules are according to the orthodox text-
books. However, the acquisition of proper co-
ordination and balance during the swing is of
fundamental importance for consistently firm
and accurate hitting. It was found that the wearing of a prosthesis to secure balance does not
seem to be essential and according to Marshall
only one member of the Society uses a prosthesis as a balancing factor (Fig. 102).

The members of the Society play off handicaps ranging from 4 to 24, which means that
any one-arm golfer who can play off 24 or less is
able to participate in his local club competitions

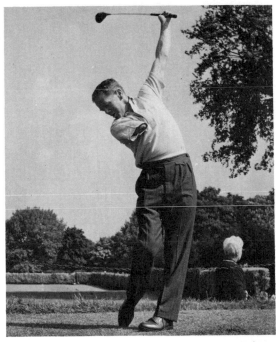

Fig. 102 Air Vice Marshal J. A. Walker, one-armed amputee playing in the Open Mixed Foursomes of the British
Limbless Ex-Servicemen Association at Roehampton,
1961.

on equal terms with normal players. The more skilled players play off a club handicap of from 8 to 14 . The most outstanding British one-arm golfer R. P. Reid, who plays off 4 handicap, some years ago won a long driving contest with a tee shot of 286 yards; a tee shot of 180 to 200 yards is considered a very satisfactory length. J. E. Watt (Sunningdale), who was a professional golfer until 1951 when he lost his right arm in a car crash, took up golf again and in 1959 was credited with 255 yards in the Society's long driving contest (indeed an excellent result of professional rehabilitation).

Skittles, Flat Green and Ten-pin Bowling

Once their equilibrium is adjusted, one-arm amputees can acquire great skill in these three sports by playing with the normal arm and can successfully compete with able-bodied players and join their clubs. Ten-pin bowling is particularly popular amongst amputees in Germany, while skittles and flat green bowling are practised more in UK. Amputees can also be trained to play with their prostheses applied to the stump; in fact, this should be encouraged, in order to promote good mobility and co-ordination in the stump as well as in the trunk. There is so far no individual data available to indicate whether and to what extent forearm amputees with the Krukenberg arm can be trained in these sports, especially bowling. This could probably be achieved only in exceptional cases, provided the player bends low enough into the crouching position to start the ball correctly and avoids damage to the stump.

Volleyball—Basketball—Badminton

Among the many ball games which can be mastered by arm amputees, the medicine ball has already been mentioned. Volleyball and basketball have become popular as team games and they, as well as badminton, are played in accordance with the accepted international rules for able-bodied players. Strict supervision is

needed, particularly in basketball, to avoid rough play (Fig. 116). Volleyball and badminton can also be played in a sitting position (see leg amputees, p. 144).

Cricket—Baseball

In Great Britain, cricket is one of the most popular games and was doubtless played by many amputees before they became handicapped. There is no reason why one-arm amputees, especially those who have practised this sport before their handicap, should not become good bowlers, provided they can adjust their posture

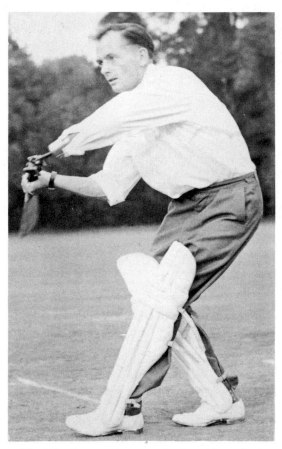

Fig. 103   One-armed amputee batting with prosthesis.

to the over-arm bowling action. Forearm amputees will, of course, have some difficulty in this respect and considerable training will be necessary, especially for high-arm amputees, to adjust their equilibrium. One-arm amputees using a prosthesis can become efficient batsmen as shown in Fig. 103, although this is an exception rather than the rule.

The same principle applies to baseball, which is a national game in such countries as the USA and Japan. There is no doubt that one-arm amputees can become skilled pitchers but the same difficulties would apply to the striker as apply to the batsmen in cricket.

Darts

The principles of dart throwing are similar to those of precision javelin throwing, and it is also a game which requires good co-ordination and accuracy. One-arm competitors playing with their normal arm can easily compete with the able-bodied in this game. Amputees with the Krukenberg arm could also train themselves and achieve skill to compete with other arm amputees at this popular pastime.

Fencing

One-arm amputees can successfully adjust themselves with their normal arm to this elegant sport in foil, sabre and épée and can join clubs of able-bodied fencers for training. In fact, for amputees who previously were right handed, this is a very useful sport for improving the dexterity of the left arm. Naturally , the acquisition of skill in this sport needs very long training, as in the case of the able-bodied fencer. The rules for fencing are those of Federation Internationale d'Escrime (FIE).

Track Events

Arm amputees can take part in virtually any form of running sport such as cross-country running, slalom, sprinting and middle and long

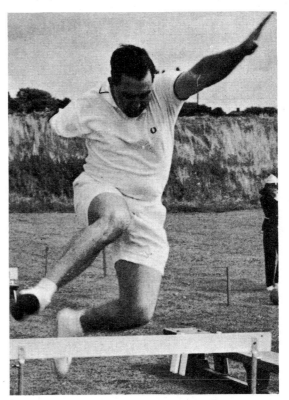

Fig. 104   One-armed amputee hurdler.

distances. The distances run in track events are 100, 200, 400, 800 and even 1500 metres. Competitors of Classes E-E1-F-F1 are allowed to run 1500 metres if it is certified by the coach that they have been trained for this event and can beat a qualifying time of 10 minutes. Hurdling is another sport practised by one-arm amputees (Fig. 104).

In order to understand the difficulties arm amputees, especially double-arm amputees, are up against during their training in running, some physiological aspects have to be considered. It must be remembered that distance runners require a high degree of cardio-respiratory efficiency for developing the necessary combination of endurance and speed. Speedy intake of air during running is essential for the rapid oxygenation of the blood, and, moreover, the oxygen has to be transferred easily from the lung alveoli to the pulmonary circulation. In sprinters, who require short-duration power to accelerate their body mass with greatest efficiency to produce maximal muscular contraction throughout short distances, the muscular work is carried out in conditions of oxygen deficiency. The oxygen debt is caused by reducing breathing to almost a complete stop during the performance, while after the event hyperventilation develops to oxydize the accumulated lactic acid and remove the carbon dioxide. In middle and long-distance running the oxygen debt will be inconsiderable during the greater part of the running, but during the final sprint the runner also decreases his respiration and consequently develops an oxygen debt. All these facts have to be taken into serious consideration in the training of arm amputees in running sports, for, as a result of the loss even of one arm, especially by high-arm amputation, but, in particular, following double-arm amputation, the muscles of the shoulder and breast girdle which are important auxiliary respiratory muscles will have suffered considerable functional impairment, with adverse effects on the ventilatory capacity of the lungs. It will, therefore, take some time before the preliminary training of amputees in running, which includes general fitness exercises, can be completed and competition training is introduced, which today consists either of formal interval training carried out on a track, or the more informal Fartlek training which takes place over the countryside, using varying types of ground. Repeated speed work over short distances and increase of pace and intensity are the principles of the controlled-interval methods by which the competitor learns to control and overcome fatigue. The resting times between the exercise periods have to be carefully considered in the competition training of one-arm amputees.

The start in short-distance running needs special mention. One arm-amputees usually prefer the low start in the crouch position, supporting themselves on the ground with the normal hand. The position of the feet, whether widespread or close together, varies and so does the position of the trunk. Decisive for a good start is the degree of extension power of the leading leg, and, therefore, the more powerful leg is placed in this position. During training, care has also to be taken from the beginning to adopt proper heel and toe running to avoid too great a stress on the Achilles tendon, which may result in its partial or complete rupture. Double-arm amputees, especially high ones, prefer to start from the standing position.

Jumping

It is generally accepted that great enjoyment can be derived from jumping events among able-bodied athletes, and it is understandable that both arm and leg amputees who were engaged in this sport before amputation are often very anxious to resume this sport and regain their skill in spite of their handicap. In contrast to leg amputees (the hazards of jumping in this type of physical handicap will be discussed later) jumping for arm amputees can be physically satisfying and beneficial, provided a thorough knowledge of the proper technique is gained and the correct building-up training is practised intelligently. Great attention has to be paid to minor details to ensure that no essentials in the training are missed. It is bad policy to practise jumping without heel spikes, because for a good jumper the action must begin from the heel of the take-off foot. To avoid bruises to the heel, a piece of sponge rubber should be put inside the shoe.

In practice, two types of jump are suitable for arm amputees; high and long jump.

High Jump. This jump is practised with run-up, either with or without prosthesis. Arm amputees are advised to use the straight jump, as the danger of falling on the stump is less than in the Western Roll and Straddle. However, double fore-arm amputees can at least be trained in the Western Roll. The bar or the line should not be raised until the arm amputee has mastered the

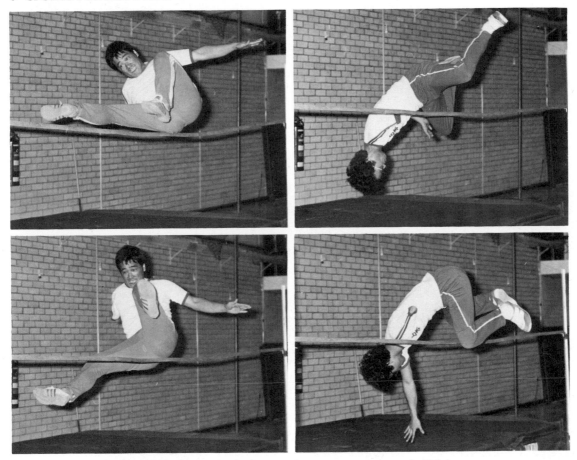

Figs 105 *Left* & 106 *Right:* One-armed amputees competing at the high jump.

control of his posture from the take-off by appropriate 'heel-ball-toe' action and adopted the proper position of his body to allow the take-off leg to give the correct upwards drive. Before using short runs, the jump should be practised from the standing position, swinging the leading leg as high as possible. Using a short run during further practice, the take-off should occur close to the bar or line so that the athlete jumps up rather than forward. This is the more essential for arm amputees, especially double-arm amputees, as their counterbalance with their stump is inefficient. To improve performance the high jumper must have very strong legs and trunk, but also be flexible in the hips; therefore, weight-training exercises, such as high kicking and trunk and hip suppling exercises, should be a regular feature of his training. Figures 105 & 106 show various techniques adopted by one-arm amputees during high-jump competitions at the first Hetero-Disabled World Games held at Stoke Mandeville in September 1974. At the 1975 Hetero-Disabled Games a Japanese one-arm amputee cleared 1.65 m in the high jump (Fig. 106).

Long Jump. Classes C and D competitors

jump with run-up, whilst those in Classes C1 and D1 jump from a standing position.

Three main styles of flight are practised in the long jump; sail, hang and hitch-kick, the simplest of which, for the beginner, is the sail. It remains to be seen whether some arm amputees, who before their physical handicap were skilled long jumpers, may ever regain such good co-ordination as to be able to achieve competitive skill in the hang and hitch-kick methods.

The basic training consists of running 5 to 7 paces and without using a take-off board jumping high, keeping the body vertical and landing on both feet. In the sail method the same technique is used as for basic training but the landing occurs on the take-off foot. After the leading thigh is driven upwards at the take-off, the knee is extended and the jumper lands on the leading foot bringing up the take-off leg to the leading leg.

Skating—Skiing

Skating is suitable as a rule mainly for those arm amputees who before their amputation had achieved some skill in this sport. Even so, the change of balance resulting from the amputation makes this sport hazardous because of the danger of additional injury resulting from a fall. For double-arm amputees, even those who were skilled skaters before amputation, this sport is not recommended and the same applies to one-arm amputees who did not practise before their amputation. Therefore, skating is limited to a very small number of arm amputees.

Skiing has become a popular winter sport for one-arm as well as double-arm amputees in countries such as Austria, Czechoslovakia, Finland, France, Germany, Norway, Poland, Sweden, Switzerland and Yugoslavia, especially for those who were skilled skiers or mountaineers before their amputation, but it is only recently that amputees in Great Britain have started to take up skiing. Unilateral forearm amputees prefer to use a ski stick fixed by a special grip to the prosthesis, while some one-arm amputees, especially those with high amputation, decline to wear an artificial arm as they feel hampered in their movements. Bilateral arm amputees have to adjust themselves even more than one-arm amputees to a new scheme of posture by training in skiing without any support. A point of disagreement amongst arm amputee skiers is whether to swing to the normal side or to the side of the amputation. However, it would appear that the majority prefer to swing to the side to which they were conditioned before amputation.

The rules of the Austrian Sports Association for the Disabled (ÖVS) apply to Alpine Skiing, Norwegian rules to Nordic Skiing. These rules have been adopted by ISOD.

Rules for Alpine Skiing Contests

(a) The course selected for the races must cause no danger to the competitors; it must not overtax the strength of the average skier nor expose him to injury. The decision on whether these conditions obtain is the responsibility of the referees for amputees, as nominated under ÖSV rules.

(b) In order to comply with the requirements laid down for amputee skiers, the following conditions govern the type of course and how it should be prepared.

Unduly flat, steep or undulating country must be avoided. The routes must be carefully prepared, so that breakage of the ski crutch device is impossible, and there must be no cause for considerable lateral swings. Soft racing areas increase the danger of accidents so they must be avoided for amputee competitors. The course must be finally tested immediately before the participants start, to make sure there are no sharp bends.

(c) The route must be so arranged that every competitor in each amputee class should be able to move freely. Sharp corners are forbidden. In order to cover the special requirements of amputee skiers, the advice of an experienced amputee skier should be sought, both when possible courses are being considered and on the choice of the actual course. A reasonable active amputee skier who has entered for the race should also be asked to advise on the choice of course. The final decision rests with the Technical Committee.

(d) Grand Slalom. The width laid down for the course must be at least 10 m. Height difference about 250–350 m.

Number of goal points: about 30 to 40, including starting and finishing points.

The width of each goal point must be at least 6 m and the distance between the posts marking two successive goals must not be less than 7 m.

(e) Slalom. Difference in height: 120–150 m

Number of goals 40 to 50, including starting and finishing points. The goal width must be at least 3.5 m and the distance between two goals must be not less than 1 m.

(f) Order of starting. The various classes of amputees will start in order of incapacity, with the least incapacitated starting first.

(g) Arrangement of the Contests. The skier must cover the course, using skis and crutch-supports.

He must complete the course without support, using only his skis, or without skis, using only his two crutch-supports. No help of any kind is permitted.

A contestant using crutches going through a goal must cross the line between the goal-posts with one foot and also his crutches.

(h) Competitors with particular qualifications may be specially placed.

One-arm amputees are restricted to only one ski-stick. Double-arm amputees who cannot use ski-sticks must, therefore, manage without them.

In the Nordic type of skiing the distances are as follows:

One-arm below-elbow amputation
    individual 8 km
    relay 4×8 km

Double-forearm amputation
    individual 4 km
    relay 4×4 km

Amputation of one forearm and one forefoot
    individual 6 km
    relay 4×6 km

Amputation of one upper arm and front portion of one foot
    individual 6 km
    relay 4×6 km

Pirogoff and one forearm amputation
    individual 6 km
    relay 4×6 km

Pirogoff and one upper arm amputation
    individual 6 km
    relay 4×6 km

Amputation of one forearm and one lower leg below knee
    individual 4 km
    relay 4×4 km

Amputation of one upper arm and one leg below knee
    individual 4 km
    relay 4×4 km

Pentathlon

Pentathlon competitions are also very popular with both arm and leg amputees. The following competitions are held:

Amputations of one forearm (including below-elbow) Class C1 (formerly E & E1)
    (a) Time required: at least two days
    (b) Disciplines:
    1. Track racing — 400 m
    2. Shot put
    3. Distance javelin throwing
    4. Long Jump
    5. Free style swimming 50 m

Amputation of both forearms Class D (formerly F)
    (a) Time: at least two days
    (b) Disciplines:
    1. Track racing — 400 m
    2. Kicking the football (distance)
    3. Kicking the football (at goal)
    4. Long jump (standing start)
    5. Free-style swimming 50 m

Amputation below elbow both sides Class D1 (formerly F1)
    (a) Time: at least two days
    (b) Disciplines:
    As in Class D but Free-style swimming only 25 m

Amputation of one forearm and one upper arm
    (a) Time: at least two days
    (b) Disciplines:
    1. Track racing — 400 m
    2. Kicking the football (distance)
    3. Kicking the football (at goal)
    4. Long jump (standing start)
    5. Free-style swimming 25 m

Amputation of one forearm and one foot
    (a) Time. at least two days
    (b) Disciplines:
    1. Throwing the club (distance)
    2. Shot put
    3. Discus
    4. Precision javelin throwing
    5. Free-style swimming — 50 m

Amputation of one forearm and Pirogoff amputation
    (a) Time: at least two days
    (b) Disciplines:
    1. Throwing the club (distance)
    2. Shot put
    3. Discus
    4. Precision javelin throwing
    5. Free-style swimming 50 m

Amputation of one upper arm and one front part of foot
    (a) Time: at least two days
    (b) Disciplines:
    1. Throwing the club (distance)
    2. Shot put
    3. Discus

  4. Precision javelin throwing
  5. Free-style swimming 50 m
Amputation of one forearm below elbow and one thigh
  (a) *Time*: at least two days
  (b) *Disciplines*:
  1. Throwing the club (distance)
  2. Shot put
  3. Discus
  4. Precision Javelin throwing
  5. Free-style swimming 50 m
Amputation of one upper arm and one thigh
  (a) *Time*: at least two days
  (b) *Disciplines*:
  1. Throwing the club (distance)
  2. Shot put
  3. Discus
  4. Precision javelin throwing
  5. Free-style swimming 25 m

Football-Tennis

This special game for amputees is played by two teams of 4 players and 2 reserves on a rectangular playing field divided into two equal parts by a cord 1 metre high.

Composition of teams

Three players with double amputations of forearm or upper arm and one with upper arm amputation on one side or a player with lower and upper arm amputations.

The Playing field

The playing field is 20 m long by 8 m wide and is divided, as mentioned above, by a centre line. Side and centre lines must be clearly marked on the ground and form part of the field and any ball which touches them remains in play. The cord, 1 m. above the centre line, should be loosely in position. A soft volley ball is used.

Rules

Each team has the task of propelling the ball, using foot, thigh, head or chest, but must not touch it with arm or hand which would be counted as a fault, out of its own court over the line into the opponents' court, until an incorrect stroke is made which ends the rally. The players must make every effort to send the ball over the line in such a way that their opponents will find it difficult to return without breaking the rules.

The ball, as it comes from the opponent, must be returned either as it bounces, or directly while it is in the air. Neither the players nor the ball must touch the cord or the posts. The return stroke does not count if the ball leaves the field of play before touching the ground. If the ball touches roof or walls, this counts as a penalty.

Passing the ball in play: (1) the ball can be struck only once by the same player; (2) it may not be struck more than three times in all; (3) before being struck, it must touch the ground only once.

If two opposing team members strike the ball at the same time and cause it to touch the line, this does not count as a fault. Another service must be made by the team which has last served.

Evaluation

(a) Each fault counts as one advantage to the opposing team.
(b) The team which has made the fault must serve next.
(c) The winning team is the one which has secured most points during the time allotted for the match. If the number is equal the result is a draw.

Umpires and Linesmen—Scorer, Timekeeper.

1. Each game will be controlled by one umpire with 2 linesmen. There must also be a scorer and a timekeeper.
2. Before the start of the game, the umpire must satisfy himself that the field has been marked out correctly and all accessories are in order. His responsibility is to declare the start and finish of the game. He is also entitled to interrupt it. He must ensure that the rules are complied with, and be prepared to give an impartial answer to all questions which may be raised.

It is the umpire's responsibility to warn a player because of rough play or incorrect behaviour, and he may order a player off the field. The umpire's position must be outside the field of play and he must announce clearly every point scored.
3. The linesmen stand at the end of each side line facing each other. They shall assist the umpire in his task.
4. The umpire blows his whistle three times to indicate that the game has begun, ended or has been interrupted. A single whistle must mark each fault and resumption of the game. The linesmen indicate a fault by raising a flag.

LEG AMPUTEES

For competitive sport by leg amputees, full adjustment of the whole person, both physically and psychologically, to the lost limb and to his artificial limb is essential. This can only be achieved by systematic training from the start.

The training of the leg amputee is divided into two parts:

Preparatory Training of the Stump

This should start as soon as possible after amputation while the patient is still in bed. The following physiological objectives should be pursued.

1. *Prevention of contractures.* It is important to instruct the patient before the amputation in the correct posture he should adopt and the exercises he must carry out after the operation. It is, therefore, essential that the nursing staff, who work in concert with the physiotherapist, must be absolutely familiar with the proper positioning of the amputee after operation. The stump should lie flat at pelvic level in extension and adduction to prevent flexion and abduction contractures. The patient is encouraged to lift his buttocks by forcing down with his hands.

2. *Adjustment of the stump to pressure.* As soon as the stitches are removed and the suture line is satisfactory (10–12 days after amputation), pressure bandages with gradually increased pressure are applied to the stump using crepe or light elastic to control oedema and to allow the amputee to become adjusted to tolerating the pressure from the prosthesis. In due course the bandage should be firmly applied 3–4 times daily and removed only during the exercise period. The technique of applying a pressure bandage varies according to individual preference but care must be taken to decrease the pressure proximally to prevent a tourniquet effect. The formation of a roll of fat above the bandage must be avoided as this, if it persists, may later give rise to friction from the prosthesis.

3. *Strengthening of the remaining muscles.* As far as possible, inactivity of the remaining muscles should be avoided from the start. In mid-thigh amputations in particular it is important to strengthen and overdevelop the extensor muscles which control the extension of the artificial knee. Special attention must also be paid to strengthening the adductor muscles as they will have been deprived of half their insertions at amputation. This results in overaction of their antagonists, the abductor muscles, especially the gluteus medius, bringing the stump into abduction. Resistance exercises by extending and adducting the leg against pressure of the hand of the physiotherapist, and later against weights and pulleys, should be carried out as often as possible.

4. *Co-ordinate movements of the stump — balancing exercises on the normal leg.* The remaining part of the thigh, deprived of the weight of the leg, has to be adjusted to a new scheme of co-ordination of the stump in relation to the hip joint. This is achieved by rotating and balancing exercises in which such simple games as kicking a soft ball can be included. As soon as the patient is out of bed, balancing exercises on the normal leg in front of a mirror are introduced to develop and maintain a good equilibrium of the body and these are followed by walking exercises on long or elbow crutches. The patient is immediately made conscious of the need to avoid tilting the pelvis. Furthermore, hopping exercises for short distances may be added. The sport which can be introduced in this period is swimming, which helps tremendously to restore balance and promote good activity of the stump. Ball games such as balancing a medicine ball with the stump, and volley ball, can also be very helpful in promoting good balance, activity of mind and team spirit.

5. *Stump hyperpathia (phantom sensation).* Following amputation, the distal part of the stump often remains hypersensitive to pressure and even to light touch. Moreover, any movement of the stump may be very painful. This discomfort is caused by adhesions which develop between the peripheral ends of the divided nerves in the stump of the amputated limb and the remaining cutaneous and muscular tissues. This irritation can become particularly troublesome if the stump has been neglected and contractures have developed. Massage and in particular early passive and active movements of the

stump in all directions can prevent it, or at least reduce the irritation to a minimum. The hypersensitivity is usually associated with a phantom sensation, ie. that strange sensory abnormality of continued persistence of the amputated part of the limb. Phantom-limb sensation after amputation may in itself be painless; it gradually lessens and may disappear into the stump in time. This is the usual development if the stump, following amputation, has received proper care and is not complicated by infection and development of neuromas, ie, formation of tender end-bulbs of the divided nerves. It is beyond the scope of this book to go into detail of the proper treatment of this condition, which consists of conservative as well as surgical procedures, but among the conservative measures early activity of the stump has proved most beneficial.

Training with Prosthesis. *(Standing and Walking)*

Surgeons, physiotherapists and limb-fitters have to work as a team to integrate the various techniques of training into a co-ordinated system to achieve the amputee's maximum skill. Before the training starts, a thorough examination of the prosthesis in relation to posture is of primary importance. The prosthesis should be worn by the amputee when it is still unfinished, as only by wearing it for some time will faults become apparent. Once he has become accustomed to a faulty prosthesis and has adopted a faulty gait it is difficult to convince him that this is due to a fault in the prosthesis. As a first step, the amputee must learn the proper technique of applying and taking off the prosthesis. This is particularly important for double leg amputee above the knee, where it is preferable to train self-application of the prosthesis first in a lying and later in a sitting position. An incorrectly applied prosthesis leads to discomfort, which complicates matters, particularly as the beginner is often unable to distinguish whether this discomfort is due to the incorrect appliance or to hypersensitivity of the stump. Some discomfort is inevitable in the beginning, until skin and

muscles of the stump adjust themselves to their new task. Further adjustment exercises in a standing position on a wall bar or between two chairs should be carried out to promote correct balance, and the position of the body in relation to the joints of the prosthesis must be maintained in such a way as to control the forward motion of the gait. From the primary standing position, various exercises are carried out which include changing the position of the trunk, changing the weight of the body from one leg to the other, lifting one leg, bending the trunk forward and backwards, and rotating the trunk and pelvis. A special exercise to develop a new scheme of postural sensibility in the stump, in relation to the movement of the foot of the prosthesis, has been recommended by Rost (1954). The prosthesis is flexed at the knee and slowly moved forwards along the floor without leaving it, and this is combined with alternating lifting and lowering the frontal part of the sole and heel of the shoe. These alternating movements give rise to different afferent impulses in the stump and eventually lead to a better awareness of the movements of the prosthesis and thus to its harmonious integration with the rest of the body. The amputee must learn to stand on the artificial leg by lifting the normal leg first for a moment and then for longer periods until he is able to stand on the artificial leg without support and with the normal leg flexed to a right angle at the hip and knee joints. Standing exercises should be carried out first in front of a mirror and later with the eyes closed.

Special attention must be paid to the training of double-leg amputees to stand unsupported. It is obvious that, even for below knee amputees, free standing takes longer to learn than in the case of one-leg amputees, who can shift the body weight to the normal leg, thus relieving pressure of the body weight from the stump and prosthesis. The double amputee carries his body continuously on both stumps, which results in discomfort and early fatigue. Above-knee amputees are trained to stand first in unfinished short prostheses, followed later by half-length prostheses until balance and endurance are developed sufficiently to allow them to stand on prostheses of normal length. Standing exercises are carried out between parallel bars, where the double amputee learns to overcome his fear of falling by standing with his arms raised forwards, sideways and upwards. This is combined with tilting and rotation exercise of the pelvis.

Once the equilibrium in a standing position is satisfactory, walking exercises are started. In this connection, it must be remembered that in the normal leg afferent impulses arise from the sole during walking, producing proper orientation in space and resulting in appropriate contractions of the muscle groups adherent to the ankle knee and hip joints and suitable associated movements of the upper limbs, which guarantees correct posture of the body during walking. These afferent impulses are missing in the amputated leg, and it takes some time for sufficiently strong afferent impulses to develop in the stump to control and neutralise the abnormal posture of the body resulting from the amputation. The untrained above-knee amputee tends to maintain his balance by compensatory movements of the trunk towards the side of the amputation on the one hand and the increased activity of the normal leg on the other. The higher the amputation above the knee, especially if it affects the hip joint, the more pronounced are these compensatory movements, resulting in a more or less marked scoliosis of the spine. Therefore, it is important in the early stages of walking exercises to avoid overstrain and fatigue. A further point which must be remembered from the start is to avoid and counteract the overaction of the abductor muscles of the leg resulting from the weakness of the adductor muscles following amputation, which is accentuated by discomfort resulting from pressure on the adductors and the whole pubic area by the prosthesis. The result is a faulty gait in abduction and circumduction.

Walking is first carried out within parallel bars, preferably with a mirror in front and another behind the patient, and, as in the case of the paraplegic, the new scheme of postural sensibility is developed gradually under visual guidance and the amputee learns to walk with the prosthesis in adduction and at the same time to avoid abnormal posture of hip and trunk. Once this is achieved and the amputee is able to control and neutralise abnormal posture, walking exercises in parallel bars with closed eyes should follow before he takes up walking with the aid of elbow crutches and sticks, until eventually free walking without any support is possible.

For the development of a correct and as near as possible normal gait, careful consideration has to be given to the correct length of the prosthesis as well as to the length of the elbow crutch and stick. A prosthesis for the above knee amputee which is more than 1 cm shorter than the normal leg leads in due course to deformity of the pelvis resulting in scoliosis of the spine. The shorter the prosthesis the more marked the development of deformity and scoliosis. It is true that a shorter prosthesis facilitates walking over uneven ground, but, as a rule, proper training should enable the amputee to negotiate unevenness of the ground satisfactorily.

A stick is only of help to the amputee for relieving weight, preventing fatigue and promoting good posture if its length corresponds properly to the height of the amputee. Too long a stick eventually causes alterations of posture and deformity of pelvis and spine.

Once the amputee is accustomed to walking on even ground he is trained to cope with various movements necessary in connection with daily activities. This is particularly necessary for an above-knee double amputee. Purposeful exercises such as sitting down on a chair and getting up from the chair, picking up objects from the floor, sitting on the floor and getting up from the floor, getting up and down stairs, walking from the pavement to the road, walking from a hard surface on to a soft surface such as grass and vice versa, walking over obstacles, are all activities which, to the below-knee amputee or one above-knee amputee, do not present too

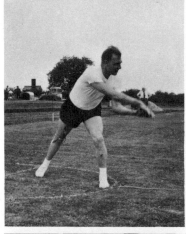
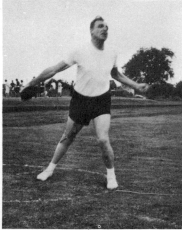
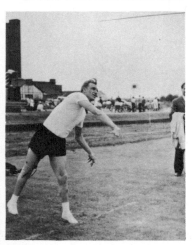

Fig. 107 *Above*: Demonstration of discus throwing by a leg amputee.

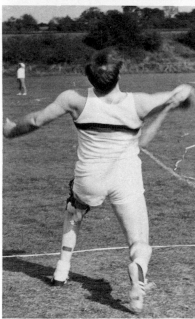
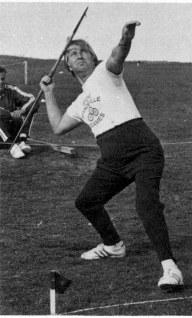

Fig. 108 *Far left*: Leg amputee throwing the club.

Fig. 109 *Left*: Action of a leg amputee throwing the javelin.

great a difficulty. They are, however serious obstacles to the double-leg amputee and can be mastered only by systematic training with the aid of two sticks and later with one stick. As mentioned above, one difficulty in the rehabilitation of amputees is the fear of falling. Therefore, exercises should be included to teach the amputee a proper technique of falling without injuring himself.

The Geriatric Amputee

The chapter on amputees would not be complete without mentioning geriatric amputees. These are people whose leg amputations, were caused by cardiovascular disease such as atherosclerosis in elderly people, diabetes or thromangitis obliterans (Bürger's disease), mainly in middle-aged people. An analysis of this group of amputees published by D. C. Welsh and R. Helsby (1973) shows that two thirds of 4,200 major amputations of the lower limbs carried out in 1968 were for patients suffering from ischaemia due to atheroma. Ninety per cent. of male patients interviewed preferred the simplicity and comparative lightness of their pylons, because for them function was more important than aesthetics in the design of artificial limbs. On the other hand, female patients (one-eighth of the total number interviewed) considered function to be as important as aesthetics. Many problems are involved in the treatment of these patients, including angina due to coronary artery abnormalities, breathlessness on effort and easy fatigue. In these patients, therefore, their circulatory dysfunction dictates the type and speed of walking training, and exercise is carried out as far as tolerance permits. Moreover, some geriatric amputees cannot use their prostheses and may need the use of a wheelchair. The scope for sporting activities in this group of amputees is therefore very limited, and as a rule only a few patients may be able to take part in them. No statistics are available on the sporting activities of geriatric amputees.

Competitions and Rules

Most of the sporting activities of leg amputees are identical to those of arm amputees with, naturally, adaptation to their specific physical defects. Like arm-amputees, they are grouped into various classes.

Field Events (Light Athletics)

Discus, club, shot-put, javelin, (both distance and precision) are practised in competitions by classes A, A1, G and B1. These classes represent single and below-knee and single above-knee amputations, including the combination with forefoot and Pirogoff amputations. These sports are carried out by single amputees with or without prostheses. Double above-knee amputees may prefer to carry out these sports without protheses and, therefore, are permitted to sit in a wheelchair.

The rules are those given in earlier chapters. Figs. 107–110 show various field-event competitions.

Archery and Dartchery

All single-leg amputees and their combinations are eligible for these sports in the standing position, while double above-knee amputees, like paraplegics, are permitted to compete from a wheel-chair.

The distance in dartchery for Classes A1 and B1 (Fig. 111 & 112, p. 142) is 8 m; for all others it is 10 m.

For details of the rules see the sections on archery and dartchery in Chapter 5.

Fencing

Competitions (individual and team entries) take place for Foil and Epée. International rules apply as described for the Stoke Mandeville Games, especially for double-leg amputees in wheelchairs.

Swimming

Classes A, B, G and G1, H and H1 should start in the water, as poor balance causes false starts. These are single below-knee amputations and their combinations. The same applies, of course, to all double-leg and thigh amputees.

Events

Breast Stroke, Back Stroke, Butterfly and Freestyle, each 100 m for classes A, B, C, and their combinations. Individual Medley 4×50 m (FINA Rules, ie. Back, Breast, Butterfly, Freestyle) except D1, Breast, Backstroke,

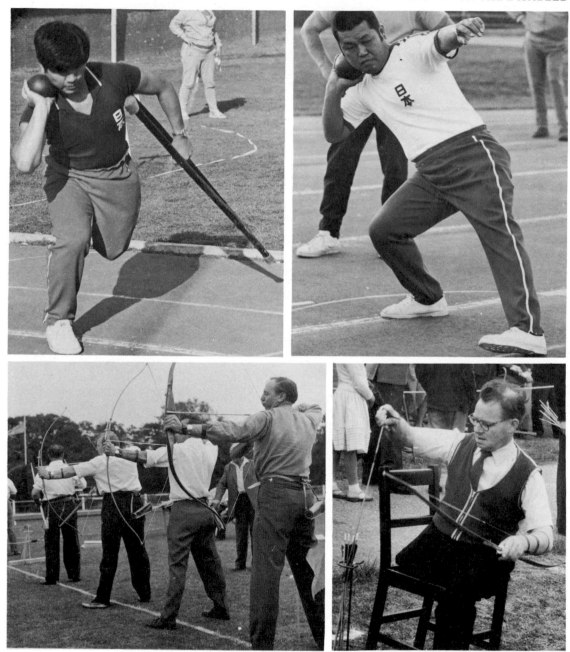

Fig. 110 *Top l & r*: Leg amputees demonstrate different shot-put techniques. Fig. 111 *Lower left*: Leg amputees in an archery match. Fig. 112 *Lower right*: High leg amputee archer competes in the sitting position.

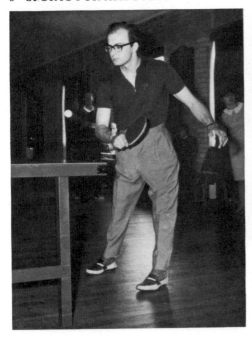

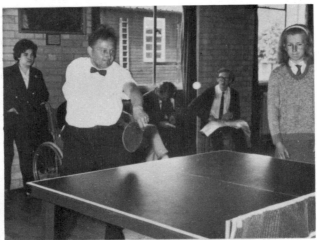

Fig. 113   A double-leg and one-armed amputee playing in a table-tennis match.

Butterfly and Freestyle each 50 m and Individual Medley 3×50 m.

Table Tennis

Competition (individual and team entries) for all single-leg amputees and their combinations are carried out in a standing position. Double above-knee amputees may play in wheelchairs. The international Table Tennis rules apply to all (Fig. 113).

Track Events

Walking and Running
The distance is 100 m for all leg amputees.

High Jump
Class B = single above-knee amputation with run-up and with or without prosthesis.

Long Jump
Class A = Single distal leg amputation includ-ing combinations, and Class B = Single AK amputation from stand without prosthesis. Classes A1 = distal lower leg amputations, and B1 = double BK and double AK, should not compete at long jump.

Pentathlon

Events for *Classes A and B*: Shot Put—Discus — 100 m   Run — 100 m   Swimming — Long Jump.
Events for *Classes A and B1*: Shot Put — Discus — 100 m   Walk — 100 m   Swimming — Precision Javelin.

Small Calibre Shooting

Competitions in this sport are carried out in standing, sitting and lying position. Club and Regional competitions have been held in some countries. It is contemplated that the first inter-national competition will be held in 1976 at Toronto during the Olympiad for the Disabled.

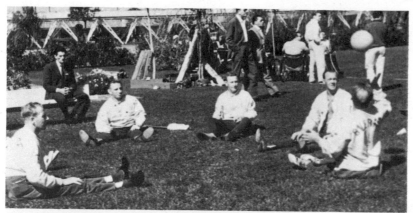

Fig. 114   Leg amputees playing sitball.

Fig. 115   Volley ball match of leg amputees.

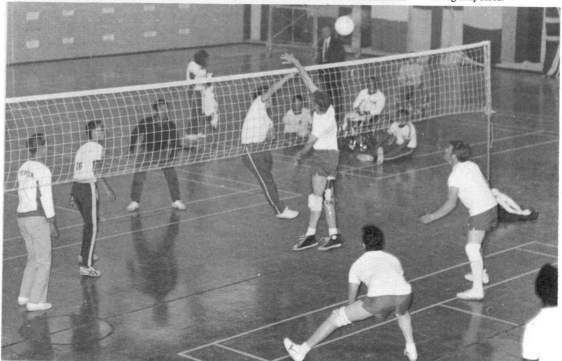

Volleyball – Basketball

These two sports can be carried out by double above-knee amputees in a sitting position (Sitball) (Fig. 114). All other classes compete in these sports standing and running with their protheses (Figs. 115 & 116).

Skating — Skiing

As previously pointed out, skating is not a popular sport amongst arm or leg amputees and is reserved mainly for those below-knee amputees who, before their amputation, were skilled in this sport. However, on taking up this sport

Fig. 116 *Right & below*:
Basketball competitions for leg
and arm amputees.

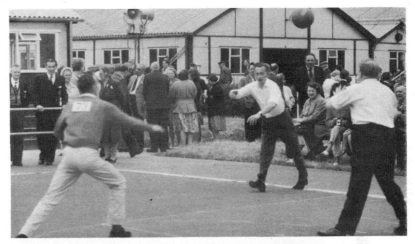

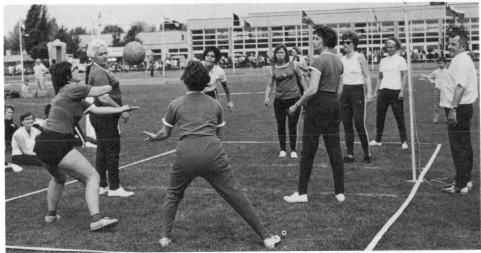

again they will at first have to exercise great caution, until they have achieved a new pattern of co-ordination and postural sensation in their prostheses. This applies, in particular, to figure skating.

In contrast, skiing has developed into a very popular sport with leg amputees, including unilateral high above-knee amputees, especially in all European countries. This sport is practised by leg amputees either with or without a crutch-ski, the former being used by both single and double amputees. In the section on skiing for arm amputees, mention has already been made of skiing by combined arm and leg amputees, and that National and International competitions have been held under both Alpine and Nordic rules. However, it must be stressed that Alpine skiing for amputees is not without danger, and fractures of various parts of the body, including clavicular fractures, have occurred. It is therefore the responsibility of the organisers to select appropriate sites for the

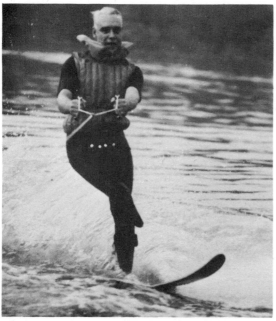

Fig. 117   Single leg amputee water skier.

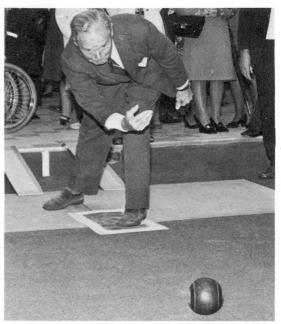

Fig. 118   Group-Captain Douglas Bader bowling the first wood at the opening of the Lady Guttmann Indoor Bowls Centre.

Fig. 119   Leg amputees playing in a skittles competition.

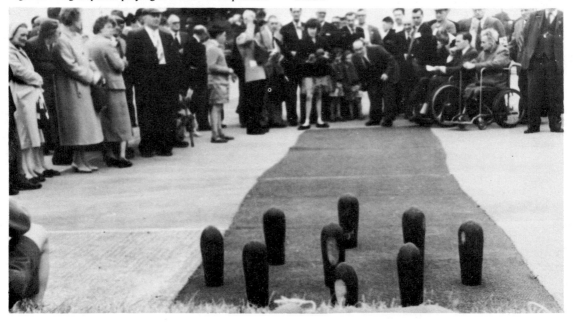

slaloms, and competitors according to their physical handicap, fitness and skill.

Mountaineering and Rock Climbing

While mountaineering has been practised by both leg and arm amputees for many years, the climbing of steep mountains is very strenuous for any leg amputee and demands systematic training. Rock climbing is even more hazardous, but the author is aware that it is practised by a very few below-knee amputees who were skilled in the sport before their amputation. Unless they are so skilled amputees should, as a rule, abstain from this sport.

Rowing, Canoeing, Sailing, Surf-Riding, Water-Skiing

While rowing, canoeing and sailing are practised by leg amputees, either with or without protheses, surf-riding is a pretty hazardous adventure sport for single-leg amputees and is, as a rule, practised only by a few who were skilled at it before amputation. Fig. 117 shows a one-legged water skier.

Skittles, Tenpin Bowling, Flat Green Bowling

These sports are practised by many leg amputees, both single and double-leg amputees of any type and also combined with arm amputation (Fig. 118 & 119). The rules are the same as those given in the section on arm amputees. Figure 118 shows Group-Captain Bader bowling at the opening of the Lady Guttmann Bowling Green.

Golf

Single and double below-knee amputees have little difficulty in playing a good game of golf, but even above-knee amputees, at least those with a single amputation, can enjoy this game by using a special technique (Fig. 120). Mention has already been made of Group-Captain

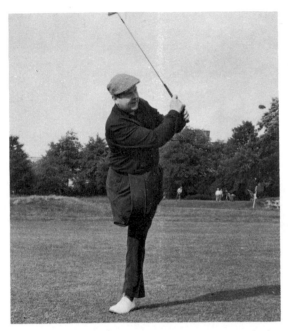

Fig. 120   Mr. Geoffrey Pain, a one-leg amputee, playing to a handicap of 5 without the aid of a prothesis, during a BLESMA Golf competition.

Douglas Bader, a single below and single above-knee amputee, who has found golf an excellent sport and plays off a handicap of six. It is worth while to quote his own experience "When I first started this game I used to swing the club very fast and fell over every time, but after a bit I discovered that swinging slowly and gripping the club lightly enabled me to keep my arms clear of my body and therefore avoid upsetting my balance. I still overbalance occasionally, but so does everybody else! Only on rare occasions does one get a stance, for instance in the left hand corner of a bunker, which is more difficult for a disabled man than an ordinary chap, the reason being that you cannot take weight on your above-knee when it is bent."

Horse Riding

Although this is not a popular sport amongst

amputees, it has been practised for many years even by double below-knee amputees. Single below-knee amputees have hardly any difficulties. Lorenzen, himself a below-knee amputee, has enjoyed horse riding for many years. He recommends for the prosthesis a somewhat larger riding boot which can be easily opened and closed by a zip, a rather ingenious idea. I remember a farmer with a single-leg amputation many years ago in my grandparents' village, who used to ride over his fields without a prosthesis, the construction of which, in those years long before the First World War, would have been too cumbersome. Leg amputees tend, when riding, to deviate toward the normal side at the trot, canter and gallop, which they have to learn to overcome. Amputees have even taken part successfully in tournaments.

Cycling

Single- and double-leg amputees, both below and single above-knee, have learned to ride a bicycle. Those who were skilled before learn to adjust themselves to the new conditions, and for those, especially, who are not familiar with this conveyance, in particular young adults, it is a good form of exercise to help them regain and improve their equilibrium. In these days of heavy traffic, it is advisable that amputees should use this type of transport only on safe roads.

TABLE 20. Records achieved by amputees at the First Hetero(Multi)-disabled World Games, 1974.

FIELD EVENTS

Javelin

Class A	41·65 m	Zajaczkowski, *Poland*
Class B	37·36 m	Sur, *France*
Class C	46·78 m	Beez, *Germany*
Class D	47·40 m	Okamura, *Japan*

Shot Put

Class A	13·2 m	Josfiak, *Germany*
Class B	11·21 m	Poplanski, *Poland*
Class C	13·90 m	Beez, *Germany*
Class D	12·01 m	Braet, *Belgium*

Discus

Class A	40·93 m	Nikkinen, *Finland*
Class B	42·10 m	Poplanski, *Poland*
Class C	46·32 m	Beez, *Germany*
Class D	39·65 m	Braet, *Belgium*

TRACK EVENTS

High Jump

Class C	1·50 m	Kraus, *Poland*
Class D	1·65 m	Okamura, *Japan*

100 m Run

Class C	10·7 sec	Kraus, *Poland*
Class C1	12·2 sec	Villozolo, *Spain*
Class D	12·3 sec	Okamura, *Japan*
Class D1	13·5 sec	Pevey, *France*

100 m Walk

Class C	28·1 sec	Hiltonen, *Finland*
Class D	24·4 sec	Hanafie, *Indonesia*
Class D1	40·6 sec	Noda, *Japan*

SWIMMING

25 m Back stroke

Class D1	22·20 sec	Perry, *France*

25 m Breast stroke

Class D1	22·01 sec	Perry, *France*

50 m Breast stroke

Class A	39·1 sec	Biela, *Poland*
Class A1	1 min 14·0 sec	Parvzel, *Poland*
Class B	47·3 sec	Kuge, *Austria*
Class B1	1 min 08·0 sec	Fujitoki, *Japan*
Class C	43·7 sec	Jaakeainen, *Finland*
Class C1	53·01 sec	Magnet, *Austria*
Class D	40·0 sec	Hillebrandt, *Holland*

50 m Back stroke

Class A	38·1 sec	Eyrd, *Sweden*
Class A1	1 min 01·9 sec	Niebur, *Germany*
Class B	45·4 sec	Grinninger, *Austria*
Class B1	45·2 sec	Bakz, *Holland*
Class C	51·1 sec	Itzhak, *Israel*
Class C1	56·8 sec	Magnet, *Austria*
Class D	49·9 sec	Lah, *Jugoslavia*

50 m Butterfly

Class A	32·2 sec	Lindstrom, *Sweden*
Class B	44·1 sec	Grinninger, *Austria*
Class C	43·3 sec	Jaaskeainen, *Finland*
Class C1	58·3 sec	Magnet, *Austria*
Class D	50·6 sec	Gasperini, *France*

Class A: *Lower leg amputation.*
Class A1: *Double below-knee.*
Class B: *Single above-knee.*
Class B1: *Double above-knee*

50 m Freestyle

Class A	30·7 sec	Biela, *Poland*
Class A1	59·2 sec	Parvzel, *Poland*
Class B	32·9 sec	Grinninger, *Austria*
Class B1	41·9 sec	Bakx, *Holland*
Class C	34·6 sec	Jaaskeainen, *Finland*
Class C1	54·0 sec	Magnet, *Austria*
Class D	34·2 sec	Hillebrandt, *Holland*

100 m Multi-stroke

Class A	1 min 15·0 sec	Biela, *Poland*
Class B	1 min 36·6 sec	Plaza, *Spain*
Class B1	1 min 56·0 sec	Bakx, *Holland*
Class C	1 min 37·4 sec	Jaaskeainen, *Finland*
Class C1	2 min 00·9 sec	Magnet, *Austria*
Class D	1 min 35·7 sec	Hillebrandt, *Holland*

Class C: *Single below-elbow amputation.*
Class C1: *Double below-elbow.*
Class D: *Single above-elbow.*
Class D1: *Double above-elbow.*

Sports for the Blind and Partially Sighted

Psychological Reaction to Blindness

Knowledge of the psychological condition of blind people is important for both the medical and para-medical attendants as well as for the physical educationalist and coach. How then do people react to their blindness? This naturally depends on whether the blindness is congenital, or has occurred in early childhood, or whether it affects individuals who have already formed their world picture by sighted education and were engaged in work and employment before becoming blind. Furthermore, it depends on whether blindness occurred suddenly through an accident or war injury or gradually following degenerative or inflammatory disease, vascular processes, tumour, glaucoma or cataract. Naturally, as in all other severely disabled, it depends on the personality of the afflicted. To most people the fear of blindness is worse than the blindness itself.

Special mention must be made of traumatic lesions. One has to distinguish between traumatic blindness produced by injury of the eyeballs and optic nerves themselves and those which are associated with brain lesions such as damage to the frontal lobes, associated injuries with the damage to the chiasma, or posterior lobe injuries affecting the inner of the posterior lobes (calcarina).

Traumatic blindness is often accompanied by traumatic shock, which cushions and numbs consciousness and makes clear thinking impossible. It may take days and even weeks before the blinded person fully appreciates the magnitude of his disablement. There exists a parallel to the psychological effects of other severe disabilities, as was discussed in the chapter on spinal cord injuries. These anxieties are of great variety and concern disfiguration, fear of losing love, loss of orientation in space, education, losing or finding employment. All this may result in losing activity of mind, despondency, despair, frustration and depression on the one hand and rebellion against one's fate and resentment against society on the other, accompanied by an unco-operative and negative attitude towards treatment and social reintegration. Interesting descriptions of the state of mind of the blind due to war injuries in their acute stages, as well as later during the stages of readjustment, have been published in Sir (later Lord) Ian Fraser's book *Conquest of Disability* (1956). He himself, blinded in 1916 in World War I and for many years until his recent death, the Chairman of the St. Dunstan's Organisation, gave a most vivid description of the adverse psychological reaction which may follow in the wake of acute blindness and how this can be overcome by 'mind over matter' (European Seminar of the Blind, 1950).

Welfare Services for the Blind

Blindness is certainly one of the severe disabilities, with the oldest and most developed welfare service organised by individuals, voluntary organisations and state legislation. In 1328 'A Shelter for 100 Blind' was established near London Wall and the Poor Law Act of 1601, passed during the reign of Elizabeth I, made it a duty of the community to provide for the blind and others unable to work. The first organised attempt made to train the blind in the United Kingdom was the foundation of a training school started by the blind poet Edward Rushton in 1791 at Liverpool. In France, the philanthropist Valentine Hauy founded in 1798 the first school for the blind (Institute Nationale de Jeunes Aveugles).

With the development of industry in the middle of the 19th century, voluntary organisations set up workshops for the blind and in 1868 Dr. T. R. Armitage founded the British and Foreign Association for Blind, now the Royal National Institute for the Blind (RNIB), whose great efforts brought the Braille System in literature and music into general use in Great Britian. The Blind Persons Act of 1920 made Local Authorities responsible for the rehabilitation of the blind and the Disabled Persons Employment Act of 1944 was a great incentive for the industrial and professional resettlement of the blind, and also of other severely disabled persons. According to statistics of the Department of Health and Social Security (Statistics and Research Division, VI, 1974) there are in England 136,146 registered blind and partially sighted persons, of whom 89,141 are totally blind.

Among the many voluntary organisations which developed after the two World Wars with the great increase in the number of the blind, St. Dunstan's Organization for Blind Ex-servicemen and Women, founded after World War I, should be mentioned, for it was this organisation which, with the RNIB, included sporting activities in its rehabilitation programmes.

Aims of Sport for the Blind

It must be remembered that blindness as such, unless it is associated with other disabilities, such as amputations or injuries of the peripheral or central parts of the nervous system, does not affect the general fitness of the individual. However, there are some specific changes of the normal pattern of movement of blind individuals, both young and adult, which include loss or decrease of free movement in space, mainly due to fear of falling or crashing against hard objects, leading to stiffness of posture, hyperlordosis and protrusion of the abdomen, and a shuffling gait. Children without early physical education are unable to perform simple and co-ordinated associated movements with their hands. They have difficulty with their physical development which results in deformities, the more so as they prefer sedentary activities which, in adult life, lead to excessive weight.

The aims of physical education and sport are, in the first place, to encourage and promote the development of readjustment forces in the nervous system, in particular the sense of orientation in space. It is well known that the trained blind acquire readjustment mechanisms in their auditory-labyrinthary apparatus and in their postural control system by developing an increased sense of touch and muscle and joint sensibility to compensate for the loss of visual afferent and efferent impulses which normally are responsible for orientation in space. In teaching free and co-ordinated movements and early sporting activities, walking, running in a straight line over gradually increasing distances, bowling and swimming are most helpful in this respect. Psychologically, sporting activities undoubtedly help the blind person to come to terms with his inner tensions and bring him out of his isolation. They bring him a new frame of mind with self-confidence, competitive spirit, contact with his fellows and, eventually, with the world around him. The more emphasis laid in the early stage of blindness on free physical training and various sporting activities the more will the blind person continue with sport as recreation for his well-being later when he is at home and in employment. Naturally, it will be easier to convince those who have had practical experience before their blindness of the value of sport than those who have had no prior interest in physical exercise or sport. In this connection, it is worth while to quote from a paper by Bill Griffiths, who was blinded and lost both forearms in the Second World War and was a prisoner in a Japanese prison camp, given at the First National Conference of the BSAD held in 1973 at Stoke Mandeville Stadium

"Many people want to know why we disabled persons, and particularly blind people, trouble ourselves at all with competitive sports. We can't hope to achieve the same results as able-bodied people—little likelihood of ever becoming a success, in the eyes of sports journalists anyway, but when we think about it, that word 'success' is a very irrelevant term. It may well mean a top-class athlete running the mile in something under four minutes, but it can equally well mean a disabled person just completing one length of the swimming bath.

Great satisfaction can be had in just learning a new sport under professional care, thereby discovering some way of lessening or maybe eliminating one's own physical disadvantage. It's good to improve upon a previous performance. At a sports meeting, I've been very dissatisfied with my performance and that's been an incentive and challenge to do better next time, and I've practised for weeks to knock the odd inch off to do better, and when the sports have come round here it's been good to pip a colleague to the post who normally pips me to it.

Physically, sports loosen up the joints and keep the muscles strong, help us blind persons to balance much better. It enables our stouthearted, resilient friends in wheelchairs to keep the upper halves of their anatomy in good trim, and it brings about this physical feeling of well-being and it can eradicate many nervous disorders too.

I've got one friend at St. Dunstan's who, ten years ago was completely confined to a wheelchair. How he has deserted that wheelchair! Four years ago he did, in fact, complete a 1½-mile walking race. Two years ago he married one of the pretty girls he met at the sports meetings. Sports have done him a world of good.

Psychologically, it can have a profound effect. It can help us to banish many fears and frustrations."

Medical and Technical Assessment—Training

The term 'blind' covers individuals with a great variety of visual defects from total blindness to useful though greatly reduced vision. Accordingly, in the medical assessment for participation in national and international sports competitions, the individuals have to be divided into two main groups: *Group A*: individuals with total blindness, ie. complete inability to perceive light, and *Group B*: Individuals with partial blindness, ie. vision up to 3/60.

There is no doubt that individuals of Group B have an advantage over those of Group A, even if their visual function is less than 3/60. On the other hand, special consideration has to be given in both the medical and technical assessment to those, whether totally or partially blind, whose blindness is aggravated by photomas, ie. visual irritations such as flashes of light or stars, or additional damage to other cranial nerves such as the trigeminal or olfactory nerves. In these circumstances, a partially blind man is certainly more handicapped than a totally blind one without these irritations, for they affect the whole person and have adverse effects on his orientation in space. To what consequences this may lead is shown by personal observation of a man who was blinded in the First World War by a handgrenade explosion. At the first accident station the rest of his right eye was removed, but the left seemed to be completely destroyed. At first he made a very good re-adjustment to his blindness and regained an excellent sense of orientation. However, he began, in due course, to suffer from photomas (optic irritations) consisting of lightning flashes of stars and light in the left, supposedly destroyed, eye only. In addition, he also developed parosmias (olfactory irritations) on the right side only. These olfactory irritations revealed themselves as a sensation of smelling burning rubber. Under the impact of these two irritative phenomena he lost his sense of orientation, became depressed, irritable with his wife and accusing her of burning things on the stove. He gradually sank into almost complete isolation. At first, this was all considered to be hysterical but when he began to have fits of unconsciousness he was admitted under my care at the neurological and neurosurgical department of the Jewish Hospital at Breslau. At operation, which was carried out under local anaesthetic, I exposed the base of the frontal lobe of his brain and found, apart from a cyst at the base of the posterior part of the right frontal lobe, that the right optic nerve was completely atrophic while the left showed normal appearance, indicating that the retina from which the optic nerve originates was more or less intact. On electrical stimulation, first of the atrophic right optic nerve, he complained after some interval of stars and light on the left side only, but stimulation of the left optic nerve, even with weak current, immediately elicited very strong photomas of the same type as those of which he had always complained before the operation. Stimulation of the right, rather scarred, olfactory nerve elicited the same parosmia he had always had of burning rubber. The left optic nerve and right olfactory nerve were then excised. The result of this operation was highly successful and the patient was not only cured of his parosmia and photoma but he also lost his fits and, in due course, regained his good sense of orientation, and his former happy family life was restored.

Other points which have to be considered in the medical assessment for sports are additional injuries to the limbs, in particular single and double amputations, spinal paralysis and cerebral damage, and in the last whether or not the blind person is suffering from epilepsy or vasomotor disturbances. Blind individuals suffering from hardness of hearing or deafness will rarely, if at all, be able to take part in organised sport because of their inability to communicate with the world around them, although some of them have at least learned to appreciate the speech of a person, by touching the speaker's larynx and feeling its vibrations.

Last, but by no means least, the medical assessment has also to take into account the fact that some partially blind individuals may aggravate their disability and that special tests may be necessary, in cooperation with the paramedical staff, to ascertain the real nature of the handicap.

The physiotherapist and coach who are responsible for the technical assessment and training of the visually defective individual have to understand the nature of the disability of the prospective candidate for sporting activities.

They have to help him in the proper choice of sports, taking into consideration his general condition, mobility and age, any additional injuries such as loss of limbs, his personality, and his own inclination to a specific type of sport in which he is interested and in which he may have previous experience and wishes to be retrained. As the coach has to deal with various classes of visually handicapped persons, he must develop a repertoire of suitable sports for the individual classes of the blind. It can sometimes be very difficult to get the blind out of their inertia, especially in the early stages of the disability, the more so if they are resentful of their fate. Moreover, the coach has to take into account the patient's early fatigue at this stage which has gradually to be overcome by systematic training. Any progress made in the training should be generously acknowledged and rewarded, for this will inspire the blind athletes to greater effort. In the later stages of readjustment the coach has also to teach the blind sportsman his limitations to prevent the over-enthusiastic from indulging in unsuitable sports and from taking unnecessary risks. It must not be forgotten that the aim of sport for the blind, as in other disabilities, is to reduce his disability and not to increase it by irresponsible behaviour.

The choice of sport for the blind is important. On the one hand the object to be pursued is to develop strength, mobility and skill, on the other the blind person must derive enjoyment and recreation from it, as this will encourage and inspire him to continue sporting activities by joining a sports club when he has returned home and taken up employment.

Training for certain sports, among them darts, bowling, shooting, walking and running, is carried out by the blind with the aid of acoustic signalling of various types such as bells, drums, electronic devices; other sports, rowing, canoeing, tobogganing and the like can only be carried out with a sighted companion. D. Teager, Principal Physiotherapist at the RNIB, in a paper delivered at the First National Conference on Sport for the Disabled

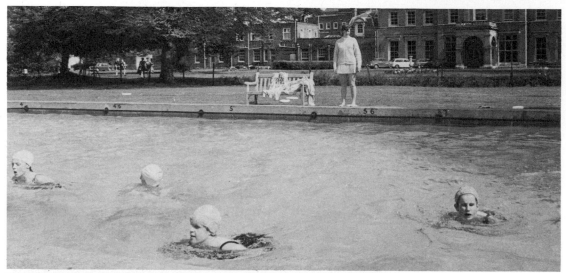

Fig. 121   Blind youngsters during a swimming contest.

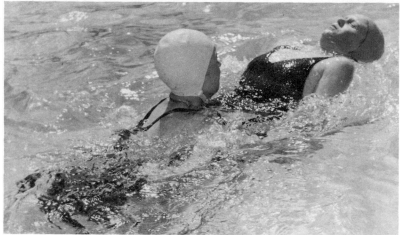

Fig.122   Life saving drill in the swimming pool at the RNIB Chorley Wood College Grammar School for blind girls.

in 1973, made some excellent points on the technical instruction to be given by a coach which may be quoted:

"The coach must be an articulate person willing to give the fullest description of technique and the correction to poor technique.

The coach must be able to demonstrate all techniques individually, if necessary breaking down complex movements into component parts. For this reason small groups or individual instruction is necessary.

The coach must constantly correct style manually (this emphasises the importance of land drill in swimming for example). However, care must be taken not to push or prod those being instructed.

The coach must demand an accepted technique for the event irrespective of the disability. I personally feel that the disabled athlete who is unable to achieve correct technique is better directed to another event where it might be possible. Poor compromises of technique inevitably

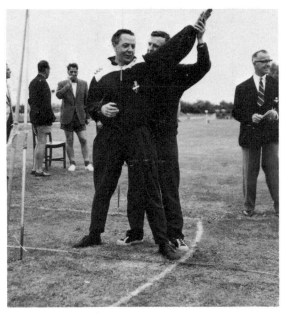
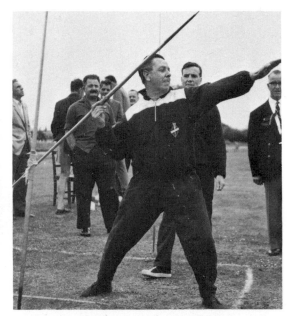

Fig. 123 *Above, l & r*: A blind athlete throwing the javelin, having been shown the direction of throw by his coach.

Fig. 124 Direction for shot put shown by the coach.

lead to low standards of performance and injury. For this reason adaptations to techniques must be carefully evaluated to fall within an accepted limit."

Competitions and Rules

Swimming

This is a sport which is very much enjoyed by the blind person for it gives him the feeling of complete freedom of movement without having to worry about direction. The training of blind children and adults in the different strokes does not materially differ from that of the sighted, but it is prolonged for competitive swimming because the blind need to learn to keep a proper course, for the splashing water and immersion of the ears may cause them to lose direction. Therefore, in competitive swimming the lanes in

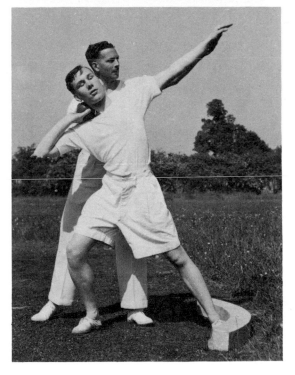

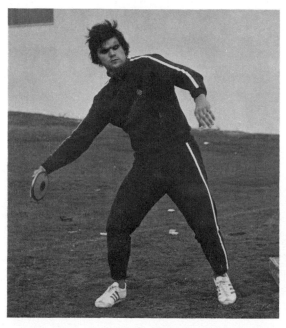 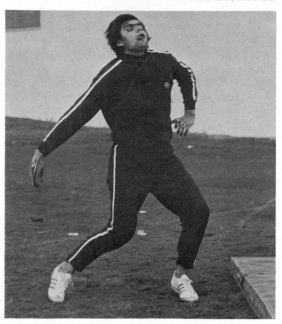

Fig.125   Blind discus thrower at the First World Multi-Disabled Games, 1974.

the water must be marked out by ropes to prevent swimming off course. Important rules for competitions are:

1. All blind swimmers start in the water.

2. Turning and finishing should be indicated by hand, and not by a stick held by the attendants a few metres in front of the finishing lane or end of the pool.

3. In relay competitions a sighted attendant should 'touch off' blind competitors and should shout a warning before the blind competitor touches to a finish or a turn in a back stroke contest. Each lane must therefore be monitored by a helper.

4. Rubber mats or other soft and well-padded devices should be fixed at the end of the pool to prevent the competitiors injuring their hands or head.

5. Competitors must not swim more than two events in each session. One hour, at least, should be allowed for swimmers to prepare for their next event.

6. Blind competitors with additional bilateral arm amputations may support themselves before the start like tetraplegics (Figs. 121 & 122, p. 154; Table 21, p. 158).

Field Events

The field events, javelin (distance), shot put, discus and club throwing have been practised by blind sportsmen and women for many years (Figs. 123–125; Table 21).

The javelin is thrown from a standing position, the discus and shot with or without spin.

1. Six competitors in each class and event should be taken forward to the final contest.

2. Once the competitor has been led into the circle he should touch the front and rear of the circle and be shown with extended arm the direction of the throw, orientate himself in space and then be left, without further instructions or assistance, to start his performance.

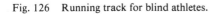

Fig. 126   Running track for blind athletes.

Fig. 127   *Right*: Blind runners: the competitor shown in the upper picture has deviated from the centre line.

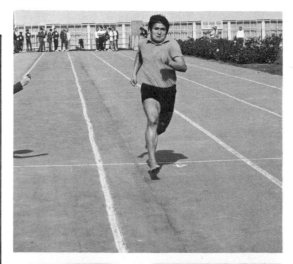

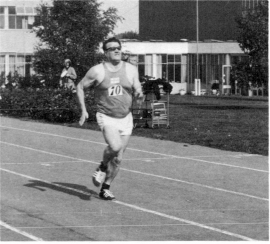

3. The rules of the FIAA apply also to the blind; therefore, if a competitor unreasonably delays making his throw he renders himself liable to be disqualified.

4. There should be an interval between events or the events should be run over several days.

Equipment Weights:

	Shot	Discus	Javelin
Men	7·25 kg	2 kg	600 g
Women	4 kg	1 kg	600 g

Track Events

1. Competitors in Class A run 60 metres, those in Class B 100 metres.

2. Competitors start on the line dividing the lanes of the track as shown in Figure 126.

3. The start is made from the centre of the track and on the line between lanes 4 and 3. The number of the starting lane is 5.

4. Competitors should be helped to read the correct starting position by a piece of tape placed along the starting line, the feel of which will enable them to position first their hands and then their feet.

The usual commands for starting the race are given. There should be a caller with a megaphone who, also on the centre line, stands facing the runner at the opposite end of the track.

5. The calling system is that introduced by the British. As shown in the diagram, the runner will be in line if he keeps on the call 5. If he moves too far to the left the caller will call 3 and the runner will know he has to move to the right. Similarly, if he moves too far to the right, the call will change to 4 and he will have then to move to the left.

Any tendency by the runner to deviate to the left or right can therefore be corrected, using this system, by continuous repetition of the numbers 3 or 4 until he runs straight (Fig. 127).

For training the blind in track events it is suggested that shorter distances, say 10, 20 and 30 metres should be attempted first, to improve their sense of direction. It is also suggested that the blind trainee should first be allowed to walk so that he can get used to the call signs; distances and speed can then be built up as he gains confidence (Fig. 127).

6. For Class B a 3 km walk with stick shall be completed, with a maximum time to be set.

High Jump

1. The high jump is competed for either from a standing position or by running up. If the back jump is used, the danger of landing on the back of the head and neck must be stressed.

2. The landing area should conform with the FIAA rule.

3. A time-limit of two minutes shall be permitted after the competitor has taken up the final start position.

4. The competitor must not touch the landing mat with his hand until the whole body has completely passed the bar.

5. If the bar is knocked off by the competitor before the final start position has been assumed, this shall not count as a failure.

6. If the bar is knocked off by the competitor after the start position has been taken, this shall count as a failure (Fig. 128; Table 21).

TABLE 21. Records achieved by totally blind athletes at the First Hetero-disabled World Games, 1974.

FIELD EVENTS		
Discus	48·91 m	Kujala, *Finland*
Shot Put	11·10 m	Kujala, *Finland*

TRACK EVENTS		
High Jump	1·50 m	Gillfors, *Sweden*
60 m Run	7·5 sec	Kozuch, *Poland*

SWIMMING		
50 m Back stroke	38·3 sec	Muirhead, *GB*
50 m Back crawl	40·6 sec	Muirhead, *GB*
50 m Crawl	32·2 sec	Muirhead, *GB*
50 m Breast stroke	46·9 sec	Aalien, *Norway*
50 m Butterfly	34·0 sec	Muirhead, *GB*
50 m Freestyle	31·9 sec	Muirhead, *GB*

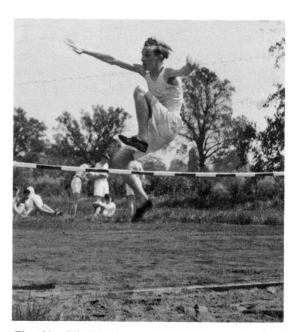

Fig. 128   Blind high jumper at RNIB Worcester College.

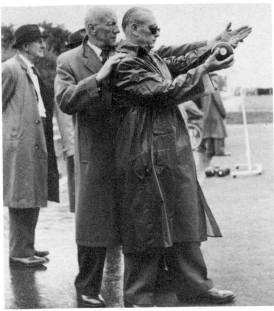

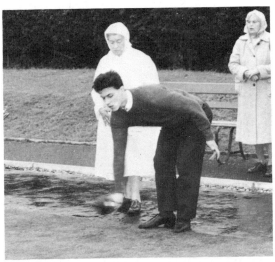

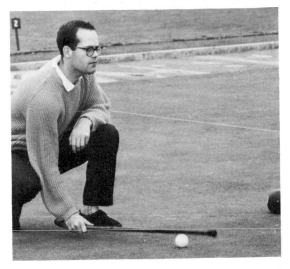

Fig. 129   *Above*: Blind bowler being shown direction of the jack.

Fig. 130   *Right upper & lower*: Blind bowler given direction by sound.

Long Jump

1. Totally blind competitors (Class A) should carry out the long jump from the standing position.

2. Competitors in Class B, ie. 0 to 1/20° vision, can compete using the run-up.

3. The take-off line shall be marked at either side by two canes painted white.

4. The landing area must be made safe.

5. Measurements shall be made from the take-off board.

6. Rules, except for those mentioned above, have to conform with FIAA.

Bowling

This is a sport where the blind can compete with sighted people and, in particular with other disabled such as amputees or the paralysed. The location of the Jack can be indicated either by holding the arm of the blind bowler in its direction (Fig. 129), by making signals such as a bell or ticking, rattling or knocking noises from behind the Jack (Fig. 130), or by a string laid from the bowling mat along the centre line of the green. The distance of the Jack is called to the bowler. The rules do not differ from those described for the sighted disabled. At one of the annual multi-disabled senior games, a blind bowler won in competition with sighted amputees and paraplegics in wheelchairs.

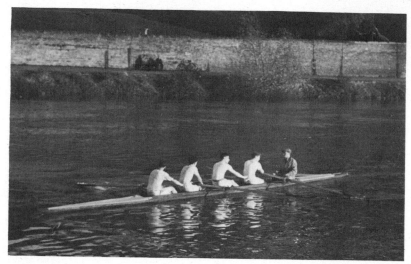

Fig. 131   A coxed four of blind oarsmen from R N I B Worcester College.

Pentathlon

1. Class A: The events are Shot Put, Discus, High Jump, 60 m Run, 100 m Swimming.
2. Class B: Shot Put, Discus, High Jump, 100 m Swimming, 100 m Run.
3. All events must be completed in 48 hours, and for Class A1 the times are laid down by the organiser.

Triathlon

1. Class A: The events are 60 m Run, Long Jump (Standing) Shot Put.
2. Class B: 100 m Run, Long Jump, Shot Put.

Rowing - Canoeing - Sailing

These sports are practised by blind people who can compete in them with the able-bodied provided they are accompanied by one sighted helper. The R N I B Worcester College for the Blind is particularly suitable for teaching rowing as it has easy access to the River Severn and the pupils achieve skill at rowing in pairs, fours and eights. Rowing instruction is started with pupils of the age of 13 years and local regattas take place between the blind crews and crews of the local grammar school. Figure 131 shows a rowing crew of four blind boys with their sighted cox (R N I B Worcester College Grammar School).

Canoeing and sailing are also suitable sports for the blind provided they have a sighted partner. The blind sportsmen must naturally be good swimmers, life-jackets must be worn, and canoes and dinghies must be fitted with buoyancy bags.

Ball Games

Several types of ball game are practised by the blind; they include football and a special ball game called Rollball. This is an interesting competitive game which is played by blind competitors in a lying position, and features in international contests for the blind on the Continent.

Skiing

The blind and the partially-sighted also enjoy skiing. Although Alpine skiing is practised,

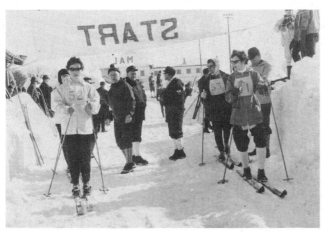 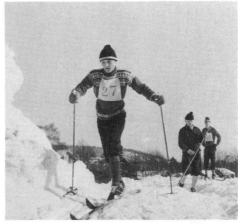

Fig. 132   Nordic skiing by the blind in Norway.

especially by those who were skilled in this sport before becoming blind, the majority prefer Nordic skiing which is certainly less dangerous (Fig. 132).

8

Sports for Sufferers from Cerebral Palsy

Terminology

The training in sporting activities of youngsters physically handicapped by cerebral palsy is as great a complex problem as is their education, training and social integration in general. Cerebral palsy is a term which embraces a great variety of unilateral and bilateral afflictions of the brain of different origin, pathology and symptomatology. It may develop pre-natally, at birth or at any age in childhood as the result of mal-development, cerebral anoxia, injuries, vascular abnormalities, infections such as viral encephalitis or meningitis, tumors and degenerative processes of the brain. The physical symptomatology is in itself of great variety and extent as revealed by hemiplegia, paraplegia, triplegia, diplegia or tetraplegia. These terms are used to describe the topographical extent of the physical defect. Hemiplegia means paralysis of arm and leg of one side of the body, paraplegia means paralysis confined to both lower or (very rarely) both upper limbs, triplegia paralysis of one arm and both legs, or one leg and both arms, diplegia involvement of all four limbs with the upper limbs less involved than the lower limbs, and tetraplegia, paralysis affecting all four limbs more or less equally. It must be noted that these terms are commonly used for complete as well as incomplete motor paralysis, although in the majority of cases the motor handicap is incomplete, ie. of a paretic rather than paralytic nature. Be that as it may, the physical handicap due to cerebral damage is usually associated with greater or lesser mental retardation and other intellectual and emotional disorders which add to the complexity of this problem.

Furthermore, cerebral palsy may also be combined with various forms of epilepsy, which may be focal (Jacksonian type) or general, consisting of petit mal, ie. short loss of consciousness only, or generalised convulsions (grand mal).

It must be stressed that there is no absolute relationship between the type and extent of the cerebral defect and the clinical symptomatology. There may be considerable destruction of one hemisphere of the brain with cyst formation (porencephaly) and unilateral hydrocephalus, as shown by air-encephalography, resulting in contralateral, practically complete hemiplegia, yet the intellectual capacity of the patient may be only little or moderately affected provided the undamaged part of the ipsilateral cerebral hemisphere and, in particular, the contralateral hemisphere remained undamaged and can develop their compensatory mechanisms. On the other hand, there may be few changes to be seen in the air-encephalogram and yet the mental abnormalities, both intellectual and emotional, may be profound due to intrinsic abnormalities of the cortical and subcortical neuronal tissues of the brain with their ramifications, dentries and glia cells.

In my own studies of cerebral palsy, which were concerned for many years with the evaluation of the anatomical brain defect in relationship to the physical and mental symptomatology as revealed by air-encephalography (Guttmann 1928, 1929), supplemented by personal observations on the exposed brain during operations for epilepsy (Guttmann 1931, 1936), I was often struck by the discrepancy which existed between the actual cerebral defect and the physical as well as the intellectual condition of these patients.

Classification

Since W. J. Little's fundamental work (1843/44, 1861, 1862) on cerebral palsy, which led to the term Little's Disease, numerous authors have suggested more or less detailed classifications of the various forms of this condition from the clinical and pathological points of view (Freud 1897; Foerster 1927; Wohlwill 1936; Phelps 1941; Perlstein 1952; Illingworth 1958; Ingram 1964; Christensen & Melchior 1967).

From the standpoint of physical education, including recreational and, especially, competitive sport, classification of cerebral palsy individuals should be made on functional considerations, including both physical and mental disability. There are four main groups to be distinguished from a physical point of view:

1. spasticity (pure or associated with rigidity)
2. ataxy
3. chorea-athetosis—dystony
4. cerebellar-atony or hypotony (atonic-astatic type)

This classification clearly reveals the inaccurate and misleading term generalising cerebral palsy children as merely 'spastics', as is commonly done by laymen.

1. The Spastic Group comprises:

    (a) hemiplegia
    (b) paraplegia
    (c) triplegia
    (d) diplegia
    (e) tetraplegia.

Spasticity may be, in its pure form, the dominant clinical symptom in all these groups, varying in intensity from mild to very profound hypertonous of the muscles with hyperreflexia, ie. the hypertonic muscle reacts to passive stretching by an initially increased resistance which relaxes by further movement. However, spasticity may also be associated with rigidity, ie. a constant muscular hypertonous with permanent resistance to passive movement in contrast to that of pure spasticity. Actually, rigidity may be so dominant that, especially in tetraplegic individuals, the whole body is held in an almost permanent, fixed and retroflexed position. On the other hand, the degree of spasticity and rigidity varies and, therefore, the pattern of movements may change as described by Plum (1958) and others. In all the spastic groups mentioned above, it depends not only on the degree of spasticity and rigidity as to whether and in what type of sport they are trainable but equally on the extent of their intellectual and emotional abnormalities.

2. The Ataxic Group

This condition consists of the inability to make rapid co-ordinated movement as a result of loss or impairment of muscle and joint sensibility. It may affect either one or both upper limbs, as revealed in the finger-nose test, or the lower limbs, as shown in the knee-heel test. In its pure form, it is extremely rare and is found mainly in individuals associated with mild or moderate spasticity. Ataxy does not necessarily exclude children from taking part in sporting activities; on the contrary, it may be improved by compensatory visual function and guidance as explained in the chapter on restoring postural control in spinal paraplegics.

3. The Athetotic-choreatic Group

This symptomatology of dis-co-ordinated involuntary movements may be unilateral, affecting mainly one arm, or bilateral, affecting both arms and legs as well as the tongue, head and neck. These involuntary movements may be associated with rigidity. In some individuals, the choreatic, in others the athetotic symptoms may be dominant. In this group of cerebral palsy, the cerebral defect is specifically located in the so-called extrapyramidal basal ganglia of the mid-brain and their nervous connections with the brain stem (caudate nucleus-pallidum-striatum complex), but sometimes the brain damage may also involve the pyramidal tracts, resulting in spasticity. Milder, especially unilateral forms of athetosis do not exclude physical education and sporting activities, the more so as intellectual disturbances may be mild or even absent, although the sometimes massive involuntary movements also affecting the speech may give to the layman the impression of severe mental involvement.

4. The Cerebellar-atonic or Hypotonic Group

This type of cerebral palsy is caused by mal-development or acquired damage of the cerebellum with its afferent and efferent connections to the brain stem and spinal cord. The symptomatology is characterised by the absence or great diminution of muscle tone and, therefore, by the patient's inability to maintain posture and keep the equilibrium of the body. On being raised from the horizontal to the vertical position the child will flop forward. As a rule this affliction is also associated with mal-development of other parts of the brain and the child is grossly mentally affected.

Physical Education and Training in Sport

The basic principle of the physical education of the cerebral palsy child is the mobilisation and utilization of all compensatory mechanisms left in the central nervous system in order to overcome the abnormal pattern of movements and posture resulting from the cerebral deficit. In the manifestation of the abnormal pattern of movements, tonic reflexes play a dominant part in the early activities of the cerebral palsy child. These reflex phenomena have been the subject of intensive physiological and clinical research (Sherrington 1913; Riddech & Buzzard 1912; Walshe 1921; Schaltenbrund 1927; Rademaker 1935; B. Bobath 1964, K. Bobath

1966; Zapella 1964; and others). The evaluation of tonic reflexes has resulted in a better understanding of the patho-physiology of the abnormal movement patterns and, indeed, has helped in the treatment and training of cerebral palsy individuals. It was found that by systematic training of these children from a very early age, a system advanced greatly in recent years by the pioneer work of B. and K. Bobath, the facilitation of normal movement patterns and postural reactions is stimulated by passive and active bilateral co-ordinated movements to counteract and overcome the abnormal reflex reactions as much as possible. The philosophy behind this modern approach to the physical education and management of cerebral palsy victims is to make them conscious and aware of the close relationship of one part of the body to the others to develop and secure control and harmony of movement patterns. Therefore, the earlier the abnormal reflex patterns of posture and movement can be checked by appropriate treatment the sooner will the child be conditioned to normal movement patterns and eventually his awareness awakened to control unwanted reflex movements. Physiotherapists familiar with this modern approach naturally play a decisive part in the training of the cerebral palsy child, which needs concentration and patience and is time consuming. Naturally, the parents, in particular mothers, have to assist the physiotherapist in her work of evolving normal movement patterns. In recent years, the Opportunity Play Groups of mothers with their abnormal children under the age of five may also play an essential part in this respect. Various sporting activities such as ball games and swimming can be included in the early training programme, and in children over five years of age many more games can be added. BSAD organizes Annual Hetero(Multi)-Disabled Games for youngsters from 8–17 years of age, in which those disabled as a result of cerebral palsy and a steadily increasing number of spastic, ataxic and athetotic youngsters, always take part.

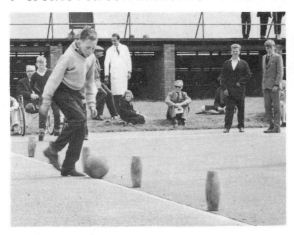

Fig. 133 Slalom by spastic cerebral palsy competitor at Stoke Mandeville.

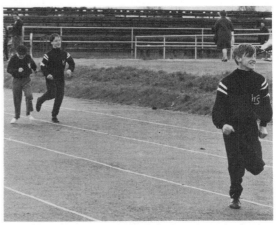

Fig.134 Spastic cerebral palsy competitors in a running race.

Assessment for Competitive Sport — Sports Events

There is no doubt that the interest in the training of cerebral palsy victims in sporting activities has increased in recent years. However, from all that has been said in the foregoing chapters regarding the complexity of this problem, proper assessment and classification of cerebral palsy participants for sports competitions still presents much greater difficulty than it does with amputees, the blind and spinal paraplegics and tetraplegics. The obvious reason for this difficulty is that the medical and psychological assessment for classification is still very much lacking as not enough of the medical advisers to cerebral palsy institutions take a real interest in the medical assessment of cerebral palsy children for competitive sport. It is therefore left entirely to the judgement of physical instructors and lay people, resulting in the grouping together of competitors of different types and levels of cerebral palsy and of various degrees of mental abnormality which make 'fair play' a farce, because according to the points system applied the most handicapped competitor will eventually be the winner of the competition in any given sport. This naturally must arouse dis-

content and frustration among competitors with lesser or minimal handicaps. As an example of an arbitrary classification, the following may be quoted:

1. minimal handicap
2. legs affected but no aids
3. arms affected
4. sticks or elbow crutches
5. paraplegic
6. tetraplegic

The first four categories are reserved for ambulant athletes and the last two (paraplegics and tetraplegics) for non-ambulant. This classification is inaccurate because (a) paraplegics and certain tetraplegics, although bound to a wheelchair, can be ambulant athletes, and (b) it ignores the different handicaps of the spastic group as compared with the ataxic and athetotic groups. Nor does it give in its general terminology any indication of the different level in the intelligence or give any indication of whether or not epileptics are included and in which games. Moreover, the definition of minimal handicap used in this classification in England by the British Spastic Society is as obscure as that of 'sub-normal' in the French classification.

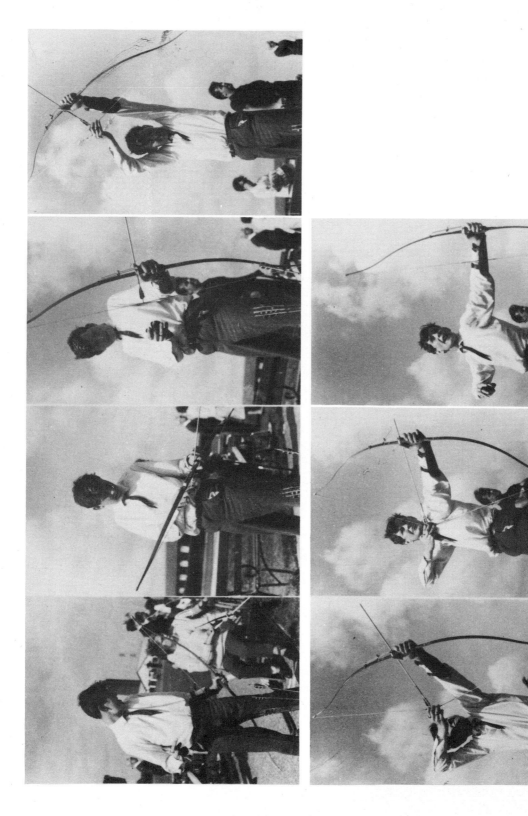

Fig. 135   Athetotic cerebral palsy archer.

Fig. 136 Training a cerebral palsy child to ride a pony.

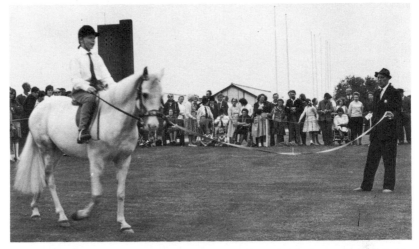

There is a great need for evaluating the classifications and rules so far adopted in various countries for competitive sport in cerebral palsy. ISOD is now preparing international classifications of the various handicaps which may clarify the rules for competitive sport in this disablement, as has been done for amputees and the blind and which ISMGF has done successfully for many years for the spinal cord paralysed.

In the Annual Hetero (Multi)-Disabled Junior and Senior Games competitions of the BSAD the following sports events are included in which groups of walking as well as wheelchair-bound cerebral palsy competitors take part: track events (walking, slalom, running relays); wheelchair dash for both hand-propelled and electric-wheelchair or tricycle users, and slalom (Figs 133 & 134). Great care should be taken in the classification of competitors for bicycle and tricycle races to avoid falls and overturns such as I witnessed at the 1975 national cerebral palsy games in France. This happened in particular in tricycle races with competitors who obviously had marked disturbances of co-ordination and had lost their balance.

Although the walking contest is an AAA walk conforming to international rules, cerebral palsy competitors are allowed to use the method of walking taught them by their physiotherapist. There is also a special free-style walk for stick and crutch users. Running competitions are only allowed for those with mild spasticity without rigidity which does not interfere, or only very little, with the isolated movement of hips, knees and feet, or those who have little impairment of co-ordination. Those with spastic triplegia, ie. considerable spastic paresis of both lower limbs and one arm, with marked adductor spasticity (Scissor gait), and those with diplegia and tetraplegia with marked adductor spasticity should be excluded from running contests.

Other sports events include archery, bowling, swimming, table-tennis, snooker, football, medicine ball, basketball, volley ball and field events. The rules applicable to these events will be found in earlier chapters. Figure 135 shows the phases of shooting an arrow, demonstrated by a young man with mild athetosis.

Swimming is an excellent and popular sport for cerebral palsy sufferers and should be started at an early age, as it helps to promote appropriate co-ordination reflexes and relaxes spasticity. However, great care should be taken with those who are suffering from epilepsy because of the danger of drowning during an attack and an attendant should be with them in the water. They should not, as a rule, take part

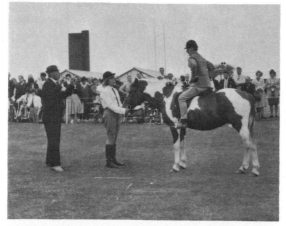

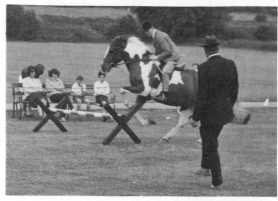

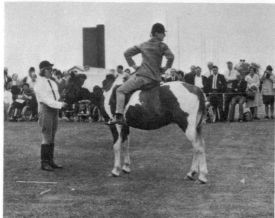

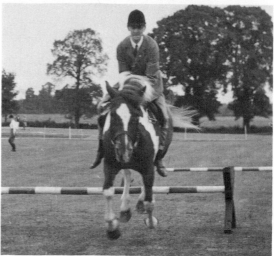

Fig. 137 *Above*: Jumping demonstration given during the Stoke Mandeville Games by a young horseman with cerebral palsy.

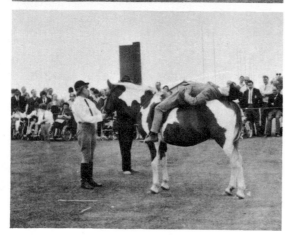

Fig. 138 *Left*: Exercises on horseback by a cerebral palsy youngster.

in competitions with those who are free from this serious complication; special arrangements should preferably be made for grouping epileptics together with special precautionary measures.

Another fundamental mistake still made in national and international cerebral palsy swimming contests is letting swimmers with considerable physical handicap compete with those of mild handicap which, of course, is unfair to the former. Conversely, by introducing a certain points system for various degrees of handicap a most seriously handicapped swimmer may be the winner in competition with mildly handicapped swimmers, which in turn is unfair on the latter and is contrary to the principles of fair play.

In recent years, training in riding for youngsters with spasticity and dis-co-ordination has been provided in various countries, and in Great Britain the Pony Riding for the Disabled Trust, a member organisation of BSAD, has pioneered this particular sport which has proved most beneficial for certain groups of cerebral palsy children. Demonstrations were given by the Riding for the Disabled Trust during the Junior Hetero (Multi)-Games of BSAD, as shown in Figs. 136–138.

9

Sports for the Deaf

As mentioned in Chapter 1, sports organisations for the deaf were set up many years before the First World War. They really are the fore-runners of the modern sports organisations for the disabled and, with the greatly improved ed-ucational and other social services for the deaf, these organisations have developed steadily in numbers and performances in many countries. Since 1924, the national sports organisations have been merged into a world organisation, the Comité International des Sports Silencieux which has so far held 12 World Games of the Deaf, the last at Malmo, Sweden, in 1973.

The British Deaf Amateur Sport Association (BDASA), a member organisation of BSAD, now has branches in all parts of the British Isles and holds various indoor and outdoor competi-tions throughout the year, including School National Athletic Championships, and National Swimming and other Sports Championships. Moreover, BDASA also takes part regularly in the World Games of the Deaf and in 1973 came 8th amongst 23 nations in stiff competition with USA, Russia, West Germany, Bulgaria, Hungary and Poland.

The standard of performance of deaf sports-men and women compares favourably with those of able-bodied national and international athletes. This is to be expected because their physical condition, as far as muscular function and strength, sensation and co-ordination are concerned, does not materially differ from that of the able-bodied, unless, as in certain cases, deafness is associated with damages to the laby-rinth resulting in giddiness and disturbance of posture, or with dumbness which makes com-munication more difficult.

Sports Events — Competitions and Rules

The sports events practised by the deaf in national and international competitions include athletics, wrestling, football, swimming, tennis, table tennis, shooting, bowling, angling, cricket, basketball, handball, volley ball, skiing, skating, snooker, long and high jump and track events. Figures 139 & 140 depict a 100 m dash for ladies and a 1500 m race for men.

The rules governing competitive sports for the deaf are those of the national and international championship competitions of the able-bodied; only a few, therefore, need be mentioned here in detail.

Snooker

(a) National teams shall consist of 3 players, Regional of 5 players;
(b) Each player shall play one frame according to the Rules of the Billiards & Snooker Associa-tion;
(c) Play shall take place on a full-sized table;
(d) The result shall be decided on the aggregate scores of each team.

Individual Championships

(a) Each game shall be one frame with the ex-ception of the final which shall be the best of 3 frames.
(b) All players must be deaf.
(c) In all competitions neither the referee nor marker shall hold the rest in his hand during the game, and it must be kept on the billiards table brackets and the player himself shall take it off when he requires it.

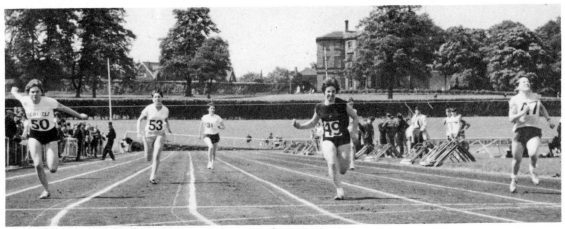

Fig. 139   Finish of deaf women's 100 m race.

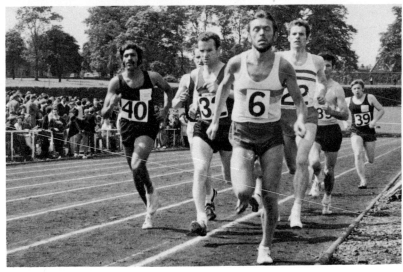

Fig. 140   Deaf competitors in men's 1500 m race.

Darts

Men's Section

(*a*) National teams shall consist of 3 players, Regional of 5 players.

(*b*) Games will be 501 up. Straight start, finish with a double. Doubles, trebles, 25s and 50s count.

(*c*) Throwing distance to be 9ft from base of board, ie. along the floor, and height of board 5ft 8in to the centre of the bull.

(*d*) A game shall consist of the best of three legs (a leg is 501 up), the toss of coin to decide who starts. Rules according to the National Darts Association.

(*e*) The inner bull, 50, is twice the outer bull, 25.

(*f*) If the number required for the game is exceeded in the course of a throw, the throw ceases and no account shall be made of any score during the throw.

Women's Section
As for men except the throwing distance shall be 8ft from base of board, ie. along the floor.

Table Tennis

(*a*) A team shall consist of three players;
(*b*) Each player shall play the best of three games against his opponent;
(*c*) The game shall be played strictly in accordance with the Rules of the ETTA.

Individual Championships
These competitions shall be organised on a national basis annually, strictly in accordance with the Rules of the ETTA.

Annual Badminton Championships

(*a*) The competition to be run according to the Rules of the Badminton Association.
(*b*) The Sub-Committee have the right to decide the date and venue.
(*c*) The BDSC have the choice of using Tourney, Official or Silver Feather Shuttlecocks according to the size of the hall where the competition is played.
(*d*) The BDSC have the right to arrange for the draw for all events.
(*e*) The Sub-Committee have the right to make final decisions regarding the seedings.
(*f*) In this competition, games are to be one of 21 points up to the quarter-finals, and best of 3 sets in semi-final and finals.
(*g*) The closing date for entries to be one month before the date of the competition.
(*h*) Players who arrive at the hall one hour after the starting time are to be disqualified.
(*j*) Players will be asked to umpire the matches, should there be a shortage of umpires.
(*k*) The umpire's decision is final.
(*l*) Players should ask the umpire first before changing the shuttlecock for a new one.
(*m*) Players to be on court as soon as their names are called.
(*n*) Players should ask the Referee of the tournament for permission to leave the hall for reasons stated.
(*o*) The Referee's decision on all matters concerned with competition is final.
(*p*) Players to wear WHITE clothes (coloured trimmings allowed).

Football

Rules
(*a*) The Football Association Laws of the Game shall apply.
(*b*) There shall be an annual Football Competition for the BDASA Trophy.
(*c*) An International Competition between England, Scotland, and Wales for the F. Bloomfield Trophy.
(*d*) Regional Knock-out Competitions for selecting players for overseas competitions.

Five-a-side Football
Five-a-side football may be played in an enclosed area, either indoors or outdoors. There are no goal-kicks, corners or throw-ins. Otherwise the rules are the same as for Association Football.

Goals	The Goals are 16ft long by 4ft high.
Goal Area	The goal area is a semi-circle of 25ft radius. A penalty spot is placed 20ft from the centre of each goal.
Ball	The ball used is size 4.
Duration	Six minutes each way; in the event of extra time being required, each team in turn is allowed a penalty. NO PLAYER is allowed to take more than one penalty.

Rules
(*a*) Only the defending goalkeeper is allowed inside the goal area and he may handle the ball only in this area.
Penalty for infringement: (*i*) by the defence, a penalty kick; (*ii*) by the attack, a free kick at the point of entry to the circle.
Note: Accidental entry by a player into the goal area which has no effect on the play is not penalised.

(*b*) Apart from this rule, there is no offside. Players may place themselves in any part of the field.

(*c*) A goal can be scored from any part of the field of play outside the goal area.

(*d*) After holding the ball, the goalkeeper must return it into play by rolling it out of his area with an under-arm bowling action. Penalty for Infringement: indirect free kick at the nearest point outside the circle to the place where the offence is committed.

(*e*) The ball must be kept below head height. Penalty for Infringement: indirect free kick at the place where the offence occurs.

(*f*) CHARGING IS FORBIDDEN. Penalty for Infringement: Direct free kick.

Schools: Boys must be under the age of 14 or 16 on the day of the competition.

Six-a-side Football (*Matches or Competitions*)

(*a*) The Laws of the Game of Association Football shall apply with the exceptions of Laws 3, 7 and 11.

(*b*) Eight players may be nominated from whom 6 shall be chosen to form a team. The game shall be played by 2 teams each consisting of not more than 6 players, one of whom shall be the goalkeeper. One of the other players may change places with the goalkeeper during the match pro-vided that notice is given to the Referee before such a change is made.

(*c*) During a game only one substitution may be made in the case of injury.

(*d*) There will be no offside.

(*e*) In the event of a match being a draw at full-time it will be decided on the basis of the number of corners gained by each side. If the match is still undecided, play will continue for a further period of 6 minutes, 3 minutes each way.

(*f*) The duration of a six-a-side game shall not exceed two equal periods of 10 minutes, except in circumstances covered by (e) above. Allowance may be made in either period for time lost through accident or other cause, the amount of which shall be a matter for the discretion of the Referee. The interval shall not exceed 5 minutes.

(*g*) The Referee shall be the sole arbiter on points of dispute and he shall be empowered to interpret the rules governing six-a-side football, bearing in mind the best interest of all parties concerned.

Exceptions

Law 3—Number of players; Law 7—Duration of game; Law 11—Offside.

Schools: Boys must be under the age of 14 or 16 on the day of the competition.

Sports Facilities for Disabled Athletes

Sports facilities for the disabled in this and most other countries are still quite inadequate to meet their needs. Although many sports centres for able-bodied men, women and children are available in every country, many, if not most of them, are unsuitable for use by the physically handicapped, especially amputees, and cerebral palsy and spinal paraplegics in wheelchairs. This applies both to sports halls and to swimming pools.

There are two barriers which make the use of many of the existing sports and recreation centres difficult and even impossible for the severely physically handicapped.

Architectural Barriers

Access to both sports halls and swimming pools is often difficult, if not impossible, for wheelchair users because of the presence of steps and stairs at the entrance to these buildings and the lack of suitable lifts inside. Therefore, unless there are negotiable ramps, and lifts large enough for wheelchair users, the disabled have to rely on the assistance of able-bodied helpers, which immediately deprives them of their independence, and may seriously affect their interest in sporting activities. Equally important is the lack of adequate toilets. Normal toilets are too small and narrow to allow a wheelchair to enter; moreover, they are often located in inaccessible places. Although in recent years municipal authorities and architects have become enlightened with regard to building houses and flats better suited to the needs of the physically handicapped in wheelchairs, the building of public sports and recreation centres, with a few notable exceptions, still lags behind in adequacy and sometimes forms insurmountable architectural barriers for double amputees and wheelchair users. In this connection it is greatly to be regretted that, unlike the Organising Committees of the Olympic Games in Rome and Tokyo, the organisers of the Olympic Games in Mexico and Munich were unable to accommodate the Olympiad of the Paralysed either before or after the Olympic Games, in spite of their most lavishly-built Olympic Stadia and magnificent accommodation for the able-bodied. This shows a lamentable lack of appreciation of the place thousands of disabled sportsmen and women have earned for themselves in the field of international sport.

The Psychological Barrier

There is another barrier to the physically handicapped in using general sports centres and, especially, public swimming pools, namely the prejudice still so deeply ingrained in society that sporting activities of the disabled are an embarrassment to the able-bodied. Therefore, if the disabled are given permission to use sports centres and, in particular, swimming pools, such permission is almost always granted with qualifications and restrictions, and thus the segregation from their able-bodied fellow men still continues. The following example may illustrate this problem. Some years ago in a certain town a new swimming pool was built and the Council gave permission for its use by disabled people on Saturdays from 6 to 8 in the evening only. However, the Council was advised by a medical officer that because some of the disabled users

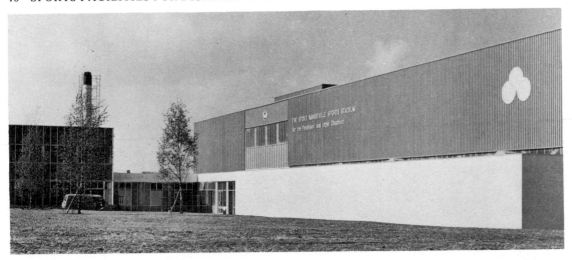

Fig. 141   The Stoke Mandeville Sports Stadium for the Paralysed. Note the three intertwined wheels of the Stoke Mandeville Games symbol on the right-hand side.

might be incontinent of urine, the strength of the chlorine in the water would have to be increased. This was done but very soon complaints arose from the able-bodied that the chlorine was affecting their eyes. The Council was about to rescind its permission to the disabled users which, in turn, would have caused dissension in the town, when one of the Council members with common sense quietly pointed out that the few incontinent disabled people would have to work very hard to compensate for the incontinence of many children and other able-bodied users of the swimming pool! Whereupon, the strength of the chlorine was reduced, the more so as the pool had continuous running water. The disabled continued to use the pool and everybody was happy!

In Great Britain under the Chronically Sick and Disabled Persons' Act of 1971 local authorities have now the responsibility for providing proper sports facilities for the disabled, by building ramps and lifts, widening doors, building proper toilets, etc., in existing sports centres and, above all, including such provisions in all new sports and recreation centres, in particular

easy access to the front door, to toilets and to all indoor and outdoor sports facilities.

The Stoke Mandeville Sports Stadium for the Paralysed and other Disabled

In view of all the difficulties just described, a new approach was made some years ago in England by the building of an indoor sports stadium specifically for the paralysed and other physically or mentally disabled persons. It was built at the author's instigation, by the former Paraplegic Sports Endowment Fund, now the British Paraplegic Sports Society, in 1968/9 at the sports ground of Stoke Mandeville Hospital under a 99-year ground lease granted by the Ministry of Health to the British Paraplegic Sports Society at a peppercorn rent (Fig. 141).

This Stadium has been designed to be completely and easily accessible to all types of disabled persons. It consists of a large sports hall, 120 × 100 ft (36.55 × 30.69 m), for games such as archery, basketball, volley ball and badminton, etc. There are smaller halls for fencing, table tennis, snooker and weight-lifting, a two-lane

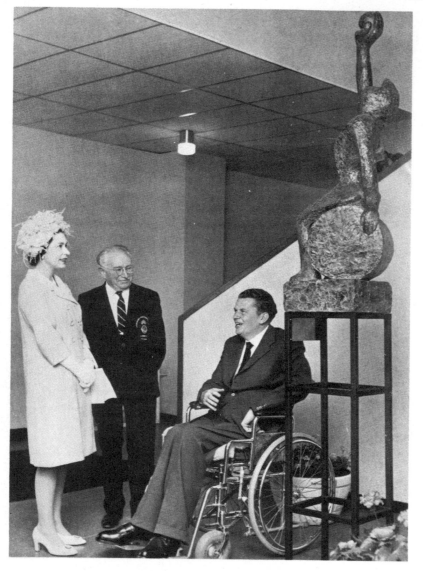

Fig. 142   HM Queen
Elizabeth II admiring the
statuette of a paralysed shot
putter and talking to Jimmy
Laird, the sculptor (wounded in
Korea, complete paraplegia
below the third dorsal
segment).

ten-pin bowling alley, a 25-metre swimming pool with six lanes and continuous running water and a large electric lift for at least 4 wheelchairs. Spectators' galleries are also included. There is a dining hall with self-service kitchen arrangements to accommodate 250 wheelchair users at a time, and, above this hall, residential accommodation for about 80 escorts, in addition to Hayward House and the six accommodation huts built outside the Stadium over the years. There is also a smaller dining room which can be used for committee meetings and, on the first floor, a coffee bar. The roomy entrance hall is connected with the administration block

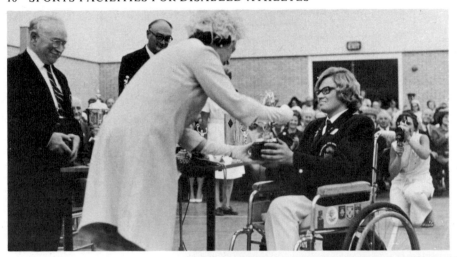

Fig. 143   *Above*: HM The Queen
presenting a table tennis trophy to
Miss Carole Bryant, MBE,
(paraplegia due to spina bifida).

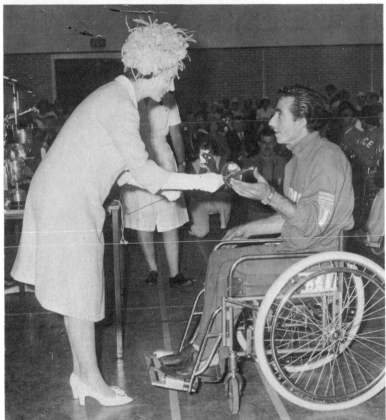

Fig. 144   HM The Queen
presenting a sword to the Captain
of the Italian fencing team.

through a desk, and the building has its own plant for the pool heating, etc. The changing rooms and toilet facilities are, of course, suitable for all types of disabled persons, including wheelchair users.

This Sports Centre for the Disabled, the first of its kind ever built in the world, was opened by Her Majesty The Queen on 2nd August 1969 on the occasion of the ISMG and has been in full use ever since (Figs. 142–144).

The Organising Committee of the Stoke Mandeville Games expresses its gratitude to the Royal Family, who for many years have taken a great interest in the sports movement for the disabled.

It was in 1958 that HRH Prince Philip attended the Stoke Mandeville Games for the Paralysed and was greatly impressed by the endurance, skill and enthusiasm of the competitors. He also opened the Second British Paraplegic Commonwealth Games in Kingston, Jamaica in 1966 and paid a special visit during the Games to the Games site, accompanied by Prince Charles and Princess Anne. Prince Philip is also the Patron of the Finmere and Northern Horse Shows, which have been organised for many years in aid of the British Paraplegic Sports Society by Mr. Bertie Allen and Miss Sally Haynes and the Earl and Countess of Swinton respectively and their committees.

Other members of the Royal Family have visited the Stoke Mandeville Games; the Duchess of Gloucester opened the Games in 1957 and the late Princess Marina, Duchess of Kent, opened the International Stoke Mandeville Games in 1966.

Once a week, paraplegic patients from the National Spinal Injuries Centre who have advanced in their rehabilitation are trained at the Stadium, and patients from the nearby mental hospital at Stone come for their twice-weekly swimming sessions. The same applies to young mentally handicapped boys and girls. Furthermore, three times a week an Opportunity Playgroup for physically and mentally handicapped

children under five is held at the Stadium which, needless to say, brings great relief to their mothers.

Annual national and international sports festivals such as the National and International Stoke Mandeville Games for the Paralysed are held at the Stadium, as are also annual sports festivals for the multi-disabled of the BSAD (amputees, the blind, and those with cerebral palsy and spinal cord afflictions), in July for children aged between 8 and 17 and in October for multi disabled adults. Moreover, the stadium is regularly used for week-end training purposes by the Stoke Paraplegic Athletic Club (SPAC) and also by the Stoke Mandeville Amputee Athletic Club (SAAC).

Although the Stadium was primarily built for the disabled, it has opened its doors also for sporting activities of certain sections of the able-bodied community, who use it daily including week-ends. Schoolchildren come every morning for their swimming lessons, and sports clubs of various types carry on their activities in the afternoons and evenings. Only during the annual national and international sports festivals is the Stadium used solely by disabled sportsmen and women.

Thus, this Stadium has made a considerable contribution in promoting a closer tie between the disabled and the able-bodied and this has helped towards a better understanding between the two sections of the community and, in particular, towards the social re-integration of the disabled into the community.

Many years ago an outdoor bowling green was built for use of the paralysed and other disabled, who competed with the able-bodied in this sport. As has already been mentioned, a large six-rink indoor bowling green was built in 1974 by the BPSS which has greatly added to the sports facilities of the Stadium and is daily in full use.

Other countries have followed our example and, in March 1974, I was invited to attend the opening of the first Sports Stadium for the Disabled in Osaka, Japan. This is a magnificent building, built on the same lines as the Stoke Mandeville Stadium following a visit by a Japanese commission to this Stadium. The next Stadium for the Disabled will be built in Oita in the South of Japan and it will probably be followed by a third in the North of Japan.

Furthermore, at the newly-opened Spanish National Spinal Injuries Hospital at Toledo, excellent indoor and outdoor sports facilities have been included. On the day this magnificent special hospital of 200 beds was opened by Prince, now King Carlos and Princess, now Queen Sophia of Spain, a National Sports Competition was held in the grounds.

11

Epilogue

I have attempted in this book to present a survey of the development of the sporting activities of the disabled during the last 30 years, but while considerable progress has been made in the sport for amputees, the blind and spinal cord paralysed, sport for cerebral sufferers and certain other forms of disability is still in its infancy. The greatest achievement during this period has been in the sporting activities of the spinal cord paralysed, considered throughout the centuries to be hopeless and helpless invalids and outcasts of society. This has really proved the powers of the human mind and spirit in overcoming one of the most profound of disablements and has revealed the tremendous readjustments forces in the human body. This young sports movement of the paralysed has achieved Olympic stature, upholding the ideals of the modern Olympic Games envisaged by their founder, Baron de Coubertin, to be free from political, racial and religious prejudices. A whole new era in sport has been opened up by the achievements of all disabled sportsmen, sportswomen and children. Many more types of disabled people, such as those afflicted by diseases of the nervous system or by muscular dystrophy or arthritis, will become more and more involved as our experience and knowledge increase. Unfortunately, society has failed so far to keep in step with the development of sport for the disabled in its duty to provide proper facilities, and the disabled are still confronted with architectural barriers and lack of understanding. Although there has been an awakening of the needs of the disabled in recent years, there is still much to be desired. I hope that this book may help to hasten this process of providing full facilities for the disabled to enable them, through the medium of sport, to reintegrate fully into the life of our community.

Bibliography

Andry, N. (1741) *L'Orthopédie, ou L'Art de Prevenir et Corriger dans les Enfants Les Deformités du Corps*. Paris

Bader, D. (1956) *I am Going to Walk*. In Frazer, Sir Ian: *Conquest of Disability*. London: Odhams, p. 147.

Bleasdale, N. (1975) Swimming and the paraplegic. *J. Paraplegia*, **13**, 124

Bobath, B. (1964) The facilitation of normal postural reactions and movement in the treatment of cerebral palsy. *Physiotherapy*, **50**, 241

Bobath, K. (1966) *The Motor Deficit in Patients with Cerebral Palsy*. London: Heinemann

Bouet (1968) *Signification du Sport*. Paris: Masson
  (1969) *Les Motivations du Sport*. Paris: Masson

Cameron, G. S., Scott, J. W., Jousse, A. J. & Botterell (1955) *Ann. Chir.*, **141**, 451

Clarkson & Maling, R. (1963) Possum. *J. Paraplegia*, **1**, 161

Colligan (1965) *Rehabilitation of the Blind*. In *Trends in Social Welfare for the Blind [Ed. Farndale]*. Oxford: Pergamon Press, pp. 274–277.

Cofer, C. N. & Johnson W. R. (1960) *Personality Dynamics in Relation to Exercise and Sport*. In *Science and Medicine of Exercise & Sport*. [Ed. W. R. Johnson]. New York: Harper, pp. 525–559

Cofer, C. N. & Johnson, W. R. (1960) *Science and Medicine of Exercise and Sport*. New York: Harper

Coubertin, P. de (1949) Les Assizes Phiiosophiques de l'Olympisme Modern. *Bull. de Comité Intern. Olympique*, **13**, 12

Cristensen, E. & Melchior, J. (1967) *Cerebral Palsy*. Lavenham, Suffolk: Lavenham Press

Diem, C. (1942) Philosophie der Leibesübungen. *Flame*, **1**, 61–69

Diem, C. (1950) *Lord Byron als Sportsman*. Cologne: Comel

Diem, C. (1957) *Sport und Alter. 18. Deutscher Sportärzte Kongress*. Frankfurt: Limpert

Diem, C. (1960) *Weltgeschichte des Sports und der Leibeserziehung*. Frankfurt: Limpert

Dietlen, H. (1926) *Herzgrösse, Herzmessmethoden, Anpassung, Hypertrophie, Dilatation, Tonus des Herzens*. In *Handbuch d. Normalen und Pathologischen Physiologie*. Berlin: Springer

Dufrenne, M. (1950) La Philosophie du Sport. *Education Physique et Sport*, **1**, 4–6

Frankel, H. (1975) Aqualung diving for the paralysed. *J. Paraplegia*, **13**, 128

Frazer, Sir Ian (1950) *Rehabilitation of the Blind*. In *Rehabilitation in England*. Thieme: Stuttgart, pp. 207–1

Frazer, Sir Ian (1956) *Conquest of Disability*. London: Odhams

Freud, S. (1897) *Die Infantile Centrallähmung*. Vienna: Hölder

Fuller, F. (1705) *Medicina Gymnastica* Lemgo

Galen of Pergamos (131–210) De Sanetate Tuenda. (Trans Green, R. M.) Springfield: Thomas

Gilliatt R., Guttmann, L. & Whitteridge, D. (1948) Inspiratory vasoconstriction after spinal injuries. *J. Physiol*. **107**, 67

Griffiths, W. (1973) *Discussion at First Conference of Sport for the Disabled*. Aylesbury: Brit. Sports Assoc. of the Disabled, Stoke Mandeville Stadium for the Paralysed

Guttmann, L. (1928) Uber einem Fall von Entwicklungsstörungen des Gehiras mit Balkenmangel (Cerebral Palsy). *Psychiatr. neur. Wschr.*, **37**, 455

Guttmann, L. (1930a) Möglichkeiten und Grenzen der Enzephalographie bei zerebrale Kinderlähmung (Cerebral Palsy). *Fortschr. Röntgenstr.*, **11**, 965.

Guttmann, L. (1930b) Die Bedeutung der Enzephalographie für die Diagnosis und Therapy der zerebrale Kinderlähmung. *Med. Klinik*, **24**, 1–4

Guttmann, L. (1931) Pathophysiologische, pathohistologische und chirurgisch-therapeutische Erfahrungen bei Epileptikern (Cerebral Palsy and Epilepsy). *Z. Neurol.*, **136**, 1–38

Guttmann, L. (1936) Röntgendiagnostik des Zentralnervensystems durch Kontrastverfahren (Air-Encephalography,

Myelography, Arteriography). In *Handbuch der Neurologie*. [Ed. O. Bumke & O. Foerster]. Berlin: Springer, **8**, pp. 187–491

Guttmann, L. (1938) Sportverletzung des. N. Thoracalis longus. *Dtsch. Z. Neurol.*, **121**, 81

Guttmann, (1945) New hope for spinal cord sufferers. *N.Y. Med. Times*, **73**, 318

Guttmann, L. (1949) The Second National Stoke Mandeville Games of the Paralysed. *Cord*, **3**, 24

Guttmann, L. (1952a) On the way to an International Sports Movement for the Paralysed. *Cord*, **5**, 3

Guttmann, L. (1952b) Olympic Games for the Disabled. *World Sport*, October Issue

Guttmann, L. (1954) De Paralyserades Olympiad. *Göteburg: Varlshorisont*, **2**, 3–6.

Guttmann, L. (1962a) *Sport and the Disabled*. In *Sports Medicine* [Ed. J. Williams]. London: Arnold, pp. 443–449

Guttmann, L. (1962b) The first ten years of the International Stoke Mandeville Games for the Paralysed. *Cord*, **14**, 30–39

Guttmann, L. (1964) The International Stoke Mandeville Games in Tokyo. *J. Physiotherapy*, **1**, 64

Guttmann, L. (1965) Reflections on sport for the physically handicapped. *J. Physiotherapy*, **2**, 252

Guttmann, L. (1967) The Stoke Mandeville Games. *Abbotempo*, London: Abbott Universal, pp. 2–7

Guttmann, L. (1967) Water therapy and water sport for the physically handicapped. *Proc. Ann. Conf. Inst. Bath Management, Blackpool*. pp. 288–289

Guttmann, L. (1969) Sport for the disabled as a world problem. (Int. Seminar, Brit. Council Rehabil. Brighton) *Rehabilitation*, **68**, 23–43

Guttmann, L. (1973a) Experimental studies on the value of archery in paraplegia. *J. Paraplegia*, **11**, 159–165

Guttmann, L. (1973b) *Spinal Cord Injuries; Comprehensive Management and Research*. Oxford: Blackwell Scientific Publications, pp. 589–599

Guttmann, L. (1974a) The value of sport for the mentally and physically handicapped: sociological aspects. *Hexagon, Roche*, **2**, 3, Part I

Guttmann, L. (1974b) *Wassertherapie und Wasser Sport für Körperbehinderte*. Congr. Intern. Soc. Badeheilkunde, Garnisch-Partenkirchen. Proceedings: *J. I. A. B.*, pp. 75–82

Guttmann, L. (1975) Development of sport for the spinal paralysed. *Hexagon, Roche*, **3**, 6

Guttmann, L. & Bell, D. (1958) In M. Hollis & M. H. S.

Roper: *Suspension Therapy*. London: Bailliere, Tindall & Cox, pp. 107–8

Guttmann, L., Munro, A., Robinson, R. & Walsh, J. (1963) Effects of tilting on cardio-vascular responses and catecholamine levels. *J. Paraplegia*, **1**, 1

Guttmann, L. & Silver, J. (1965) Electromyographic studies on reflex activity of the intercostals and abdominals. *J. Paraplegia*, **3**, 1

Hartel, Lis (1956) *As Young as Your Courage*. In Frazer, Sir Ian: *Conquest of Disability*. London: Odhams, p. 17

Henhem-Barrow, J. A. *Social Welfare for the Blind*. In *Trends in Social Welfare*. Oxford: Pergamon Press, pp. 262–273

Huizinga, J. (1949) *Homo Ludens*. London: Routledge & Kegan Paul

Illingworth, R. S. (1958) *Classification, Incidence and Causation of Cerebral Palsy*. In *Advances in Cerebral Palsy*. London: Churchill

Ingram, T. S. (1964) *Paediatric Aspects of Cerebral Palsy*. Edinburgh: Livingstone

Jochheim, K. A. & Strokendl, H. (1973) The value of particular sports of the wheelchair-disabled in maintaining health of paraplegics. *J. Paraplegia*, **11**, 173

Jonson, W. R., Hutton, D. C. & Johnson, G. B. (1954) Personality traits of some champion athletes as measured by two projective tests. *Res. quart.*, **24**, 484

Jokl, E. (1964) *The Scope of Exercise in Rehabilitation*. Springfield: Thomas

Jokl, E. (1965) Sport as Leisure. *Quest*, **4**, 37–47

Jokl, E. & Suzmann, M. (1940) Aortic regurgitation and mitral stenosis in a marathon runner with special reference to effects of valvular heart disease on physical efficiency. *J. Am. Med. Assoc.*, **114**, 467–470

Kaplan, H. (1968) *Games and Sport as Leisure*. New York.

Klein, I. W. (1847) *Gymnastik für Blinde*. Wien

Kruger, H. C. (1962) *Avicenna's Poem on Medicine*. Springfield: Thomas, p. 24

Ling, P. H. (1834) *Medizinische Gymnastik*. Upsala

Little, W. J. (1843–1844) Lectures on deformities of the human frame. *Lancet*, **i**, 5, 38, 78, 174, 285, 350, 598, 705, 809

Little, W. J. (1861) On the influence of abnormal parturition, difficult labour, etc. *Lancet*, **ii**, 378

Lorenzen, H. (1955) Schwimmflossen für Amputierte. *Arzt und Sport Suppl. Dtsch. Med. Wschr*, **80**, 638

Lorenzen, H. (1962) *Lehrbuch des Versehrtensports*. Stuttgart: Enke

Loy, J. W. (1969) The nature of sport. *Quest,* **10,** 1–15

Loy, J. W. (1970) *Soziologie des Sport.* In Grolle und Stromeyer: *Jugend und Sport.* Vienna, pp. 158–168

Lüschen (1960) Prolegomena zu einer Soziologie des Sports *Kölner Z. Sozial & Sozial Psychol.,* **12,** 505–515

Maimonides (1199): *Treatise on Hygiene*

Mallwitz, A. (1954) *Artz und Versehrtensport.* Stuttgart: Enke

Maslow, A. H. (1954) *Motivation and Personality.* New York: Harper

Mercuriale (1569–1573) *Libri VI. De Arte Gymnastica.*

McIntosh, P. (1963) Sport in Society. London

McIntosh, P. (1966) 20th-Century attitudes to sport in Britain. *Intern. Rev. Sport Soc.,* **1,** 19–30

Munro, A. & Robinson, R. (1960) Catecholamines in tetraplegics. *J. Physiol.,* **154,** 244

Parade, G. W. (1930) Herzerkrankungen und Sport. *Med. Welt.,* **10,** 1101

Parrisius, W. (1924) Ski Races. *Münch. Med. Wschr.,* **71,** 1601

Perlstein, M. A. (1952) Infantile cerebral palsy; classification and clinical correlation. *J. Am. Med. Assoc.,* **149,** 30

Phelps, W. M. (1941) Different characteristics of spasticity and athetosis to therapeutic measures; *N.Y. State J. Med.,* **41,** 1824

Plum, P. (1956) Cerebral palsy of 543 cases. *Dan. med. Bull.,* **3,** 99

Plum, P. (1958) The prognosis in cerebral palsy. *Dan. med. Bull.,* **5,** 58

Plum, P. (1962) Early diagnosis of spastic paraplegia. *Spastics Quart.,* **11,** 4.

Rademaker, G. C. (1935) *Reactions Labyrinthiques et Equilibre.* Paris: Masson

Riddoch, G. & Buzzard, E. F. (1921) Reflex movement and postural reactions in quadriplegia and hemiplegia with special reference to the upper limbs. *Brain,* **44,** 397

Salathiel, T. (1965) *Services for the Blind.* In *Trends in Social Welfare.* Oxford: Pergamon Press, pp. 253-261

Schaltenbrand, G. (1927) The development of human motility and motor disturbances. *Bull. N.Y. Acad. Med.,* **3,** 54

Slusher, H. S. (1973) *Existential Humanism and Sport.* In *Sport in the Modern World.* Berlin: Springer, p. 549

Schreber, D. M. (1852) *Kinesiatrik.* Leipzig: Fleischer

Sherrington, C. (1913) Reflex inhibition in the co-ordination of movement and posture. *Quart. J. exp. Physiol.,* **6,** 251

Talbot, H. S., Rocco, A. G. & Conroy, M. E. (1957) A Preliminary Report on Ventilation in Quadriplegic Patients. *Proc. 6th Conference Spinal Cord Injury.* American Veterans Administration, p. 20

Walshe, F. M. R. (1923) On certain tonic and postural reflexes in hemiplegia with special reference to the so-called associated movements. *Brain,* **46,** 2

Warfield, L. M. (1934) The heart and athlete: a modern concept of cardio-vascular disease. *Ann. Heart Ass.,* **3,** 5

Watson-Jones, R. G. (1955) *Fractures and Joint Injuries Vol. II.* Edinburgh: Livingstone, pp. 1019–1038

Wenkart, S. (1963) The meaning of sport for contemporary man. *J. Existential Psychiat.,* **3,** 397–404

Weiss, M. & Beck, J. (1973) Sport as part of therapy and rehabilitation of paraplegics. *J. Paraplegia,* **11,** 166

Weiss, P. (1969) *Sport—A Philosophic Inquiry.* London

Werner, I. A. L. (1838) *Medizinische Gymnastik.* Dresden: Arnold Buchhandlung (see previous literature)

Wingo, C. F. (1957) Pulmonary Ventilation Studies in Twenty Quadriplegic Patients. *Proc. 6th Conference Spinal Cord Injury.* American Veterans Administration, p. 23

Widener, K. (1962) *Erziehung Heute-Erziehung Morgen.* Zürich

Wohlwill, F. (1936) *Zerebrale Kinderlähmung.* In *Handbuch der Neurologie.* [Ed. O. Bumke & O. Foerster]. Berlin: Springer

Wolfenden, Sir J. (1960) *Report on Sport and the Community.* Central Council of Physical Recreation

Wolfenden, Sir J. (1969) Sport and the community. *Rehabilitation,* **68,** 23–27

Zapella, F. (1964) Postural reactions in 100 children with cerebral palsy and mental handicap. *Develop. Med. Child Neurol.,* **6,** 475

Zander, G. (1879) *L'établissement de Gymnastique Mécanique.* Paris: Masson

Index